Public Expectations and Physicians' Responsibilities

Voices of medical humanities

John K Crellin

Faculty of Medicine
The Health Sciences Centre
Memorial University of Newfoundland
Canada

Foreword by
T Jock Murray

Professor Emeritus
Dalhousie University

T0203453

Radcliffe Publishing
Oxford • Seattle

Radcliffe Publishing Ltd
18 Marcham Road
Abingdon
Oxon OX14 1AA
United Kingdom

www.radcliffe-oxford.com
Electronic catalogue and worldwide online ordering facility.

British Library Cataloguing in Publication Data

A catalogue record for this book is available from the British Library.

ISBN 1 85775 642 8

Typeset by Advance Typesetting Ltd, Oxford
Printed and bound by TJ International Ltd, Padstow, Cornwall

Contents

Foreword

In recent decades medical educators have recognized that the medical humanities deserve serious attention in the education of future physicians, and can't just be taken for granted. The emphasis and the majority of curricular time in medical education has been on the medical sciences and on clinical competence, with little attention and time on the humanistic aspect of medical practice.

It is perhaps not surprising that the exciting advances in medical science over the last century have captivated physicians, medical educators and the public. The advances of anesthesia, surgery, vaccines, antibiotics, pharmaceuticals and diagnostic imaging have fostered a biomedical view of illness and this has brought dazzling advances in medical treatment. But this has resulted in an increasing specialization of personnel and a technical and pharmacological approach to medical care. The training of physicians has emphasized scientific and technical competence as the essence of the modern physician. The discussion of 'medical science' made it sound as if medicine was a science, rather than a caring profession that used science as one aspect of how it attempts to prevent illness, treat disease and care for those who are suffering. And the argument also suggested we cannot teach caring, empathy and understanding of others. The 'old' idea of the humane and caring doctor was nice and it would be a happy happenstance if the new scientific doctor was also a warm, empathetic, communicative, and caring person, but these seemed to be personal qualities that we can assume and take for granted in the bright students we select for medicine. Don't we need to spend our educational efforts on the hard, ever changing and difficult medical sciences, because we can take for granted that future physicians will use their science in a caring fashion?

We hear from the public that the bright physicians who care for them are not always caring, not always communicative, not always good listeners who strive to understand the nature of the person with an illness, and who don't always seem to be acting in their best interests. The criticism of doctors is usually about their lack of humanistic qualities, not that they don't know enough science.

I think it is a truism that everyone wants an array of qualities in their personal physicians. In fact, most would not hesitate to list some of these. They usually start with a request that their physician listen to them, respect their concerns and respect them as persons. It is interesting that almost all discussions begin with a request for communication, respect, empathy and interest in them as persons, and only later in these discussions does the issue of medical knowledge and scientific competence come up, not because it is less important but perhaps because they take this for granted. It is interesting that the profession takes the humanistic aspects of the physician for granted, emphasizing scientific, clinical and technological competence, while the public and patients emphasize the importance of the personal and humanistic aspects of the physician, tending to take for granted that they are scientifically trained. They would always want a competent physician, and would reject a caring, listening physician that was not medically and scientifically competent as well.

We have often heard the question, 'But who would you rather have – a surgeon who was highly skilled in the operating room, or one who was warm and communicative and a good listener?' The question seems a reasonable one if we watch a lot of TV medical dramas, as they focus on dramatic medical events that require immediate technological competence, often by professionals who are insensitive and rude, inept as members of a team, and dysfunctional in their personal lives. That they were smart and highly competent in their scientific medicine seemed to excuse their generally unpleasant behavior. This book suggests that the question about competence or caring is a false question as we need and expect, and should demand, that they be both.

Fortunately the situation in medical education is changing, and the EFPO Project (Educating Future Physicians of Ontario) has catapulted the issue to the forefront of medical education reform in Canadian medical schools and has led to reform of postgraduate medical education by the Royal College of Physicians and Surgeons of Canada through the CanMeds Project. The idea was simple but profound. It began with the question of what qualities should characterize future physicians when they went out into practice? After long discussions with the medical profession, other health professions, governments, health agencies and the public, they outlined categories of expectations that could be translated into objectives of medical education. A physician should be a medical expert and decision maker, a collaborator with other professionals, a health advocate, a manager and gatekeeper, a life long learner, a scientist-scholar, a person and a professional. Professor Crellin shows how the humanities can be used to address these expectations in medical teaching, using resources such as literature, art, history, film, poetry and philosophy.

Medicine was always a balance of the art and the science of medicine. The medical humanities are about values in medicine. And although desired, they can no longer be taken for granted and must be a serious concern and commitment in medical education. This does not mean a de-emphasis of the medical sciences, but aims for a balanced educational philosophy that incorporates both.

On a personal note, I don't know anyone who could have written this book but John Crellin. He has a long experience in medical education and an unusual skill in teaching with a wide array of the humanities, respecting each, and as he shows in this text, recognizes what each can bring to the understanding of the human condition and to the understanding needed by the next generation of physicians. He is a respected and much published medical historian, an expert in the history of pharmacy and alternative medicine, but also one who teaches with film, works with the native community in their healing ways, and knows the recent advances in medical education and how the humanities fit into the most advanced concepts of medical education.

Despite an increasing commitment to do something about affecting the balance of sciences and the humanities, most medical schools are not sure how to incorporate the concepts fully within the curriculum. Professor Crellin provides a well written, erudite and entertaining guide that will assist every medical school.

Dr T Jock Murray OC, MD, FRCPC, FAAN, MACP, FRCP, LLD, DSc, DLitt
Professor Emeritus
Former Dean of Medicine and Professor of Medical Humanities
Dalhousie University
March 2005

Preface and acknowledgements

Public Expectations and Physicians' Responsibilities is offered to all those – physicians and other healthcare professionals and students, as well as the general public – who have concerns about the provision of healthcare. Underpinning the book is the perception that the values held by physicians have changed in recent years and may not be in keeping with the needs of patients today. Particular attention is given to the qualities that the public wishes to find in its physicians – and, by extension, other healthcare practitioners – as well as the responses of physicians. The public and professional voices found in the book are taken from an emerging field of study called medical humanities. The reasons for and the value of this approach are made clear in the introductory chapter.

The book grew out of resources developed for a course on medical humanities for medical students at the Faculty of Medicine, Memorial University of Newfoundland. Established in 1996, the course developed at a time when increasing concerns were being expressed about whether the professionalism of physicians was declining. It was thus timely that an interdisciplinary group of faculty members at the university were in favour of broadening ethics teaching to embrace, in a formal way, the co-curricular activities in the humanities that were already being offered to students.

The initial preparation of course material was aided by a generous grant from Associated Medical Services based in Ontario. This allowed students from medicine and other disciplines – Thusitha Anandakrishnan, Trina Barnes, David Baxter, Oliver Ennis, Martin Johnson, Fergus O'Brien, Susan Payne, Sarah Prabhakaran, Nancie Rideout and Keith Rose – to offer thoughts and input. Key faculty colleagues who were enormously supportive in terms of ideas and in providing time in leading small groups of students for discussion of course materials were Raoul Andersen, Bill Bavington, Pamela Hall (artist-in-residence) and Bernard O'Dwyer. Thanks are also due to Penny Allderdice, D'Arcy Duggan and Peter Harris. Special acknowledgement also goes to the Rev. Peter Barnes and to the Rev. Bill Bartlett who contributed time and insightful thoughts from their positions in pastoral care. Rosalind Nichols masterfully contributed to the project by preparing educational material, often at short notice, with equanimity and graciousness. JDC has, as in so many years, added her own unique support.

Lastly, I would like to express my appreciation for the promptness and courtesy of the staff of Radcliffe Publishing, Gillian Nineham and Jamie Etherington in particular.

John K Crellin
March 2005

CHAPTER 1

Voices from medical humanities: an introduction

The last decades of the twentieth century witnessed a striking outpouring of public concerns about healthcare. Many of these are noticed in *Public Expectations and Physicians' Responsibilities* as it considers the qualities that the public hopes to find in physicians, indeed in all healthcare practitioners. In so doing, the book draws on medical humanities. Emerging in the 1970s, this field of study explores observations, other than from the sciences, on the human condition, especially on its illnesses, suffering and values.

Medical humanities

Readers of this volume – physicians, other healthcare practitioners and administrators, patients and everyone interested in healthcare – will see at least six broad, albeit overlapping, roles for medical humanities that can contribute to quality care:

1 providing practitioners with insights into the values of patients and practitioners as well as their attitudes toward health and illness
2 prompting practitioners to reflect on the diverse needs of patients, and on practitioner–patient relationships
3 alerting practitioners to what is needed in order to provide humane care to patients
4 prompting patients to consider their own role in healthcare
5 examining the nature of medicine, and the reciprocal influences between medicine and society
6 contributing specifically to patient care settings as therapy or as healing for physical ailments, the mind and the spirit.[1]

The various roles are not mutually exclusive. Britain's National Co-ordinating Council and Centre for Integrating the Arts and Humanities into the National Health Service, for instance, believes that an 'arts on prescription' philosophy will lead to doctors having more depth and breadth in their education and to patients achieving mental well-being through creative expression.[2]

The field of medical humanities is broad, almost catch-all. Areas of popular culture, ranging from movies to 'medical thrillers' and romance novels, add to insights from such established disciplines of the humanities as literature (including the now popular genre of patients' narratives), history, ethics, philosophy and the visual and performing arts.[3] Each subject area offers particular perspectives into the human condition as it relates to health and disease.[4] Contributions also come from anthropology, folklore and sociology insofar as they draw attention to, for instance, lay beliefs and social values about healthcare.

Some people might be tempted to argue that all the necessary perspectives on lay beliefs, values and expectations can be gained from social science and historical studies alone. This, however, ignores a key role of medical humanities, namely that, unlike the emphasis in the social sciences on understanding groups, cultures and populations, it is about appreciating the *diversity* and *individualism* of patients.[5] Medical humanities questions whether a 'standard' patient exists. It has been said that literature, through focusing on particular characters and situations, reveals more fully than the trends identified by historians how changes in medical practice impact on *individual* lives; it reveals, too, 'the social realities in the dilemmas that physicians and patients alike faced in the wake of new discoveries and technologies.'[6] As an instance, John Bayley's moving account of a railway journey with his wife, a sufferer from Alzheimer's disease, reveals a pattern of difficulties familiar to all in similar circumstances. Yet, at the same time, unique to Bayley's situation was the international fame of his wife Dame Iris Murdoch, one of the influential novelists and philosophers of the twentieth century.[7] It has, too, to be appreciated that the writer, the artist, whatever form of expression he or she uses, is generally a practised observer able to look from the outside, from the margins so to speak, and to offer carefully considered perspectives.

Although this volume is not a history, the interpretations of historians about trends are included, for an important part of medical humanities is to provide context and an understanding of constant and changing lay attitudes. For this reason, although the timeframe in this book mostly covers recent decades, it forays into the first half of the 1900s and even earlier, not only to make comparisons, but also to illuminate persistent public concerns as well as to comment on, for example, current nostalgia for the old 'country doc'.

This volume introduces readers to many resources, some well known, others less so. A few lengthy quotes are included to show how the humanities illuminate individual perceptions, e.g. the happenings in a physician's waiting room or a physician agonising over his or her detachment from patients. However, this is not an anthology. The book relies mainly on references and short quotes to document a point as it *recommends* and *invites* a reading or a viewing of an entire story, a painting, or other resource.

Many public concerns about medicine spotlight ethical issues; indeed, ethicists have been conspicuous in challenging medicine since the 1960s. However, ethical analyses are not included in the following chapters because of both lack of space and the availability of innumerable ethics/bioethics texts. Nevertheless the value of medical humanities for studying ethical dilemmas becomes clear. As stressed by others, the social context commonly provided by, for instance, fictional stories underscores that, in real life, clear-cut decisions to ethical dilemmas rarely exist, only best answers.[8] Additionally, medical humanities commonly raises everyday ethical dilemmas that are given little or no attention in ethics textbooks – for instance, whether it is a physician's responsibility to provide spiritual care if so requested by a patient.

Many physicians have voiced the same concerns as the public, often resting on results from social science investigations. Although medical voices commonly stem from professional dilemmas, even disillusionment with much medical practice, they do reassure the public that some physicians are listening to their disquiet. Physicians' voices in this volume are, for the most part, taken from those expressed through medical humanities' resources, especially from novels, short stories and essays. Widespread public acclaim has come to some physicians. The renowned American poet, essayist, short story writer and physician William Carlos Williams, who continued medical practice alongside international success as a writer, said: 'I have never felt that medicine interfered with me but rather it was my very food and drink, the very thing that made it possible for me to write.' Williams' interest in people was 'right in front of me. I could touch it, smell it. It was myself, naked, just as it was.'[9] In fact, physicians have often found that creative expression, rather than writing 'standard' case histories, is needed to illuminate suffering and responses to it. Writings directed primarily to the medical profession are also culled, in part because they not only offer the public further insights into the minds of physicians, but also because they, too, indicate physicians' efforts to find words and analogies that express the complexities of suffering amid shifting values within society and medicine.

It is appropriate to notice again that the book is intended for a broad readership. The field of medical humanities has developed rapidly in recent years not only in medical schools, but also as undergraduate and graduate level courses in general university studies. The subject area and the issues raised by medical human-ities are relevant to everyone concerned about healthcare, not just the professionals involved. Lay readers can, for instance, analyse and compare their own responses to illness and expectations of medicine, consider the roles they expect of their physicians, look at their own responsibilities in healthcare, gain an appreciation of the concerns and tensions facing physicians, and, more narrowly, wonder how medical humanities can contribute to the moral order of a medical school and the development of the 'good' physican.[10]

Physician roles and the organisation of this book

It is not easy to organise the wide range of material offered by the humanities. One obvious challenge is to show how the attitudes and opinions of individuals resonate with, help to shape, or conflict with public opinion. In this book, the qualities and roles that the public expects or hopes for in its physicians offer a focal theme. Moreover, the expectations give a pragmatic focus by pinpointing issues on which the medical profession needs to respond, and certainly not to push aside as being too vague or philosophically abstract.

In developing the theme of roles, the book draws on an influential project that emerged in Canada in 1990. Following a doctors' strike in Ontario during 1986, which raised questions about whether doctors were losing traditional values and 'abandoning the covenant of service to society', Associated Medical Services established a programme called Educating the Future Physicians of Ontario (EFPO).[11] In developing the EFPO project, extensive consultations with the public and groups of health professionals were used to identify what roles the public expected of its physicians.

The roles were identified by the following descriptive names: medical expert/ clinical decision maker, collaborator, health advocate, manager ('gatekeeper'), learner, scientist-scholar, and lastly, with the input of consultations with physicians, a person.[12] These roles have, in part, been relabelled or reorganised by medical schools and organisations; for instance, at one medical school students need to be familiar with the role of 'communicator/educator/humanist/healer'.[13] Such adaptations, however, are in keeping with the spirit of the original data as is the case in this volume where being a professional is viewed as the overarching or umbrella role, as it were, to which all the other roles contribute.[14] In fact, examining public expectations as a whole spotlights the need for society and physicians to examine closely the nature of professionalism and its current – i.e. early twenty-first century – role in quality care.[15]

EFPO has gained national and international influence beyond Ontario medical schools through such medical bodies as the Royal College of Physicians and Surgeons of Canada, which developed, for example, the concept of roles in its CanMEDS 2000 programme for residents in specialty training.[16] An important issue is whether or not the Royal College's efforts to evaluate the 'skills' and 'competencies' of residents in fulfilling the roles – using agreed-upon criteria – captures the values that are part of the public's expectations of the roles.[17] It must be said that of the triptych of educational goals in medical schools – 'knowledge, skills and attitudes' – it is attitudes that are commonly glossed over, largely because of the difficulty of measuring them.[18] This volume supports the view that medical humanities offers physicians-in-training, indeed all practitioners (especially those with limited clinical experience), a sharper sense of public expectations than guidelines to issues found in such documents as the American Board of Internal Medicine's 'Project Professionalism' (discussed in Chapter 2), or from the 'attitudinal objectives' for medical students and physicians adopted in the United Kingdom.[19] Furthermore, medical humanities helps to explore the many issues raised in discussions on developing a more formal social contract between the medical profession and society than presently exists.[20]

In this volume, the roles have been divided into two parts. Part I, 'Foundation Roles', looks at public expectations that challenge individual physicians to consider their values and responsibilities to patients. Part II deals with factors that more directly shape the physician's role as medical expert and clinical decision maker. Although the latter role acknowledges public expectations of sound and up-to-date knowledge, we look particularly at how metaphors and stereotypes – disseminated widely throughout the voices of the humanities – may affect decision making. In both parts, some 'byways' are included; they serve not only to illustrate a particular theme, but also the broad scope of medical humanities and how, by illuminating the complex relationships between medicine and society, this can encourage physicians to look broadly at the society in which they work. Lastly, a short Epilogue raises questions about responsibilities and roles for patients as well as physicians in healthcare.

'Humanities are the hormones' (*William Osler*)

One particular intention of this book is to prompt reflection not only among physicians, but also other healthcare professionals. When medical humanities first gained a formal place in medical education during the 1970s, it was part of a response to calls for greater caring and compassion in physicians, and the not uncontested view that this could be taught.[21] It was felt that the more rounded the medical education, the more likely it would produce a humane or caring doctor who is both sensitive to and understands human nature in increasingly ethnically diverse societies.[22]

Support for the value of medical humanities persists despite critics who emphasise the lack of studies demonstrating that the humanities have any influence on medical practices.[23] Indeed, doubts exist over any correlation of humanistic studies with humane behaviour, just as questions continue to be raised over whether the formal teaching of ethics can produce more ethical doctors.[24] On the other hand, given that no area of education has the same influence on everyone, the weight of intuitive and testimonial support for the value of the humanities for individuals cannot be dismissed as merely 'anecdotal'. Such medical authorities as Sir Geoffrey Keynes, the Blake scholar and innovative surgeon, noted (1981) his delight in literature and in particular the life and work of William Blake; Keynes commented: Blake kept 'alive in my mind the value of imagination in a material world – an important background to a profession which might lead to a slight twist of inhumanity.' He went on to write that he liked to think that perhaps Blake contributed something to 'my attempted humanisation of the current fashion' of radical mastectomy in the treatment of breast cancer.[25] Testimonials continue to be found in the current promotion of medical humanities courses.[26]

When world-famous physician William Osler (1849–1919) stated that 'humanities are the hormones', he spoke as a wise physician and a student of human affairs. The occasion was his 1919 address, 'The Old Humanities and the New Science', delivered to the prestigious Classical Association in Britain.[27] He made the analogy of hormones ('essential lubricators for the body') to the lubricating role of humanism within society. If he were alive today, Osler would certainly see the humanities as essential for the humanism of physicians and, perhaps, essential for patient-centred care. He would probably agree with RS Downie's comment that 'healing in its many forms generates moral problems which the arts can portray through detailed narrative or with dramatic immediacy';[28] such portrayals can only prompt reflection.

Tensions in medical education

Ever since Osler's time, medical education has faced a tension between its aspirations to graduate the 'good' – when it means the humane if not the learned – doctor and its mandate to produce a 'technically' safe one. The tension, which needs to be understood by the public as well as by the profession, has been accentuated in recent decades by increased demands for practitioners to master the explosion of new information in the basic medical sciences, new diagnostic technology, countless new drugs, and the pursuit of 'evidence-based' practice. In the United States, it was observed in 2001 that a changing culture of academic health centres implicitly undermines the 'values and principles of caring that medical educators wish to impart.'[29] Emphasis on the safe doctor prompts questions about what priority is given to medical humanities courses within medical schools. Unfortunately, many students, amid the examination pressures of a curriculum, place humanities – ethics included – low in their priorities. Frustrations over the eclectic nature of medical humanities can also be an issue, perhaps more so when medical humanities programmes are a collection of separate courses leaving students to construct for themselves the key 'messages'. Hopefully, the present volume with its framework for synthesising many aspects of medical humanities responds to this.

As medical humanities explores the human condition, it must be said that its questioning tone can be unsettling for many physicians and students. Its keen eye for medicine's failures, and its questioning of physician power, can be viewed as akin to 'doctor bashing'. This can undermine not only the spirit of the seasoned physician, but also of medical students, who, prior to their clinical training, may acquire a sense that scientific knowledge offers certainty – at least from the way it is often taught. Yet uncertainty needs to be fully appreciated, just as all healthcare practitioners need to appreciate the diverse needs of patients.[30] Anatole Broyard's *The Patient Examines the Doctor* helped one reader, a medical student. She initially felt misunderstood by the author and wanted to explain to him that it is not always easy to be a 'star', to be a wise and charismatic communicator, after having worked an 80-hour week and not a soul giving a damn that you are tired or that you miss your family. 'I wanted to yell at the top of my lungs that "letting yourself plunge into the patient [and] losing your own fear of falling" [as Broyard requested] takes more courage, serenity and faith than just idealizing about it on paper.' But the student went on to feel that, if she was in Broyard's position, she might feel the same about his relationship with his physicians. 'Therefore,' she continued, 'it dawned on me that Broyard was not trying to ignore the struggles that I will face in my career. I realized that he was just trying to convey his position. He was explaining to his literary audience who he was and the perspective he had, just as he wanted to explain this to his doctors. He was not attacking me. He was revealing his soul. Just as I want understanding, Broyard wanted to be understood.'[31]

A further area of tension surrounding medical humanities, insofar as it relays many demands raised by society, is that it seems to be asking physicians not only to be humanists, but also to be 'Renaissance' people who can offer a wide range of services to individuals and to society. These include being a sensitive counsellor on innumerable topics, perhaps on complementary/alternative medicine, or praying with patients – topics often little explored in medical schools. Practitioners have justly asked, 'How can I provide all the services that are being demanded of me?' or 'Is too much being expected of me?' As one British physician wrote in 1995, the role of 'family doctors as generalists, friends and family counsellors is threatened' since they are now 'expected to function as pioneers in preventive medicine, all-round physicians, financial managers and committee members.'[32] He added that there is a real danger that patients are looked upon in both research and medical practice as 'one or more sick organs, and that the effect of disease on other systems, not to mention its impact on their lives, is neglected.' A button badge distributed by the Center for Professional Well-Being in the US, proclaiming 'I Can't Please Everyone', resonates with many practitioners and students alike who are daunted by public expectations and demands, a situation that surely needs to be understood by patients and the public in general. This book suggests that there must be a recognition that limits exist to what any one individual can accomplish within contemporary healthcare systems; nevertheless, responsibilities remain for all healthcare practitioners to ensure that patients do not suffer when inabilities exist to meet a patient's expectations or worries.

In approaching the tensions, tendencies exist for physicians to approach 'horror' stories about medical incidents – grist to public–physician tensions – by dismissing them as one-sided or embroidered. Sometimes they are, but healthcare practitioners also need to appreciate the strength and influence of critiques from well-informed journalists and academics. For instance, a 1994 social science text, entitled *Challenging Medicine*, highlights the cumulative impact of a wide range of confrontations to medicine that include nursing, healthcare management, malpractice litigation, television and animal rights advocates.[33] Such challenges, it should be mentioned, are partly fed by uncertainties within western societies, a questioning of traditional ways and institutions, and worries about the future of healthcare – all part of what is broadly termed our postmodern age.[34]

Notes on resources

> As a chronically ill patient I long to find such a doctor as Dr Hullah [in Robertson Davies' novel, *The Cunning Man*]. I have encountered the Dr Oggs [in the same novel] in my past who thought science was the ultimate example. This to me, excluding the bootlegging and general incompetence of Dr Ogg, represents the vast stream of doctors who have 'treated' me. Simply looking for a simple solution, a quick solution, and if the answer did not reveal itself: 'there is no problem.'[35]

This book is not only suitable for personal reading, but also for group discussions of the debatable issues.[36] In moving from one public wish or expectation to another, particular attention is given to readily accessible short stories, novels, essays and movies. Moreover, information on many such resources is available through the incomparable medical humanities database maintained by New York University.[37] Behind the success of the database has been the development of a sub-discipline, namely Literature and Medicine; like medical humanities as a whole, this is eclectic in scope, much more than 'medicine in the classics' – a favourite topic for many.[38]

As said, we also draw on the responses and observations of doctors – data banks of experience – in stories, poetry, essays and many other resources. The short stories and commentaries of physician Michael LaCombe are good illustrations; he is also editor of two volumes, *On Being a Doctor*, which, in combining the prose and poetry of physicians *and* patients, makes them especially notable among a number of significant humanities resource books.[39] In a contrasting way, the stories and memoirs of Richard Selzer offer striking images of medicine and patients by a surgeon who revels in the art of a wordsmith.[40]

With respect to voices heard through popular culture, a good number of movies with medical themes and depictions of good and bad doctors are cited. Experiences with showing such movies – even the 'B' movies that excel in reinforcing stereotypes – to a variety of audiences confirm the perceptiveness of George Bernard Shaw's quip that a film is educating you far more effectively when you think it is only entertaining you. Those who believe movies have little influence on patients must consider views about the impact on people who visit psychiatrists (*see* Chapter 10). Moreover, it seems clear that television medical dramas – reaching almost epidemic proportions by the end of the twentieth century – are significant sources of information about medicine, if not adding a sense of uncertainty about the medical care they receive.[41] It must also be said that movies undoubtedly help medical students and physicians stand outside the profession, so to speak, to look at the profession with the gaze of the public. All those who are not healthcare professionals can also ask themselves to what extent do their own views match those of Hollywood stereotypes.[42]

Although 'one picture is worth more than a thousand words', we can only reference a few. These include how artists interpret health and illness in their paintings – fears, hopes, the meanings of illness, and much more. Artists such as Canadian Robert Pope and Mexican Frida Kahlo are just two who hauntingly highlight the loneliness of being a hospital patient subjected to technological scrutiny.[43] Readers may be surprised that, in great contrast, twentieth-century comic postcards are often cited. In fact, as an intriguing barometer of popular culture, they offer sharp commentary on the pomposity and foibles of physicians. When postcards had their 'golden age' (c. 1900 to 1914), literally millions of them were mailed annually. Although their popularity then declined, the smaller numbers continued to comment on many aspects of social change, as they still do. The commercial success of comic cards suggests that they resonated with the mindsets of countless purchasers and serve as a more sensitive indicator of popular attitudes than many cartoons appearing in, for instance, such magazines as *Punch* or the *New Yorker*.

An understanding of popular attitudes and perceptions reveals many reactions to healthcare that physicians do not anticipate. For instance, what can be common and garden tools to the practitioner can be tellingly different for a layperson; a vaginal speculum, for instance, may symbolise the invasion of sexuality by some women, though some moderation in attitudes may have resulted since 1996 through the theatrical performances and book by Eve Ensler, *The Vagina Monologues*.[44] Distilled from the thoughts of over 200 women about their vagina, Ensler's work is not only a striking example of a public voice trying to demystify health and illness, but also an illustration of the diversity of resources for medical humanities.

The development of a physician

Whether or not the reader is a layperson, a medical practitioner, other health professional or a student, the nature of the education of a physician is a concern, especially in how it shapes values and attitudes. Resources for insights are legion. Tensions in medical education have already been noted, much of which can be seen as part of a strange journey. Melvin Konner, in his *Becoming a Doctor: a journey of initiation in medical school* (1987), wrote that medical school provided 'an unusual journey'; although not the sort of journey undertaken by anthropologists. This he described as 'a voyage into an arctic waste or a semi-arid wilderness or a dense, hot, wet tropical forest in search of human or protohuman exotica.' He added, 'I have taken that sort of journey, so I can attest that the [medical] one described here, if less romantic, is no less exotic and it is not devoid of drama and palpable danger.'[45]

There is, in fact, an extensive literature of writing about medical school and internship experiences; much of it is somewhat critical and leaves a sense of uncertainty among many lay readers.[46] Peri Klass, author of *A Not Entirely Benign Procedure* (1987), noted the therapeutic role of writing:

> As a medical student, writing gave me a voice at a time when I would otherwise have had none. As hospital wisdom goes, the medical student is on that part of the totem pole that is buried underground. I could go home and tell the story my own way, write out my revenge on people who tortured me (or surpassed me), my anguish about my own inadequacies, my reactions to the life and earth around me – and publish it. It was diary and therapy; but also, to tell the truth, power and glory.[47]

Such experiences speak to the value of students keeping journals of their experiences. These can fulfil various roles such as helping to prompt reflection on changing personal and professional values, to consider the nature of relationships with patients, and to create a narrative that helps to deal with the fragmentary and uncertain nature of medicine. Keeping a journal can thus serve as an integral part of the medical humanities education of medical students, just as a journal that is mindful of health matters can be helpful to many lay people.

Novels, sometimes indirectly, can also prompt thoughts about the development as a physician. A compelling example is Robertson Davies' *The Cunning Man* (1994). An 'autobiography' of physician Jonathan Hullah, it can be recommended as a must-read for any layperson or professional for its insights into public concerns over the comparative lack of holism in conventional medicine.[48] In another successful novel, *The Case of Doctor Sachs* (2000), physician Bruno Sachs struggles to make sense of his experiences and his questioning of medicine. Physician–author Martin Winckler wrote: 'Medicine is a sickness that strikes all doctors, in varying ways. Some derive lasting benefits. Others decide one day to turn in their white coats, because that is the only chance of cure – at the cost of a few scars.'[49] Winckler himself did just that and turned to full-time writing in 1994. Readers can justifiably ponder on the issues, the tensions and the dilemmas that lead to such decisions.

In closing this introductory chapter, we also want to make clear that, while medical humanities draws 'lessons' and 'messages' from the humanities, pedagogy should not interfere with the uplift of spirits, the flash of inspiration, the calming of the mind and the relaxation from a piece of art, an absorbing novel, a piece of favourite music – seen, read or listened to without any thought of it contributing specifically to one's education or professional life.

Endnotes

1 For comments on goals (1) and (2), Evans HM and Greaves DA (2002) 'Medical humanities' – what's in a name. *Medical Humanities Edition of the Journal of Medical Ethics.* **28**: 1–2.

2 The Co-ordinating Council was established in 1999 as a joint activity between the Nuffield Trust for Research and Policy Studies in Health Services and Durham University. For quote, oft repeated in the UK, www.studentbmj.com/back_issues/1299/news/446b. html (accessed July 2004). Various programmes in arts and healthcare have been established for a number of years, especially in the US as part of a conspicuous

arts-for-healthcare movement, led principally by the Society for the Arts in Healthcare, founded in 1989.

3   Defining the boundaries of medical humanities often occasions debate; however, the scope indicated here is well represented in writings accepted as medical humanities. Popular culture, it should be added, can be defined as the everyday world around us, ranging from the mass media to popular psychology and religion. As popular culture emerged as an academic discipline in the 1970s, it was often described as the 'new humanities'.

4   It should be added here that disquiet often arises over 'insights' from popular culture due to many pitfalls in interpretation. Stereotyping, for instance, can be so extreme as to be dismissed. However, few commentators doubt that, overall, popular culture reflects many widely held attitudes and perceptions. It is clear, for example, that movies provide important connections between medical knowledge and popular culture. For general discussion, Apple RD and Apple MW (1993) Screening science. *Isis.* **84**: 750–4; also for subtle issues of interpretation, Crawford TH (1998) Visual knowledge in medicine and popular film. *Literature and Medicine.* **17**: 24–44.

5   It must be said that the growth of interest in qualitative research in the social sciences – in part due to concerns over the type of information gathered from surveys – commonly captures individual voices that concur with many sentiments emerging from the humanities. It is appropriate to add that Downie RS and Charlton B (1992) *The Making of a Doctor: medical education in theory and practice.* Oxford University Press, Oxford, Chapter 7, offer a discussion on 'The preclinical curriculum: social sciences and humanities'. They indicate that in fulfilling the need to respond to 'whole-person' care, it must be appreciated that the social sciences are not concerned with uniqueness and, in fact, encourage detachment; the role of the humanities is in helping with the interpretation of patients' meanings.

6   Furst LR (ed) (2000) *Medical Progress and Social Reality: a reader in nineteenth-century medicine and literature.* State University of New York, Albany, p. xi. Emphasis added.

7   Bayley J (1999) *Elegy for Iris.* Picador, New York, and his other writings about his wife. For emphasis on patterns, Scott PA (2000) The relationship between the arts and medicine. *Medical Humanities Edition of the Journal of Medical Ethics.* **26**: 3–8.

8   The relationship between medical humanities and bioethics has been discussed from various viewpoints, e.g. Carson RA (1994) Teaching ethics in the context of the medical humanities. *Journal of Medical Ethics.* **20**: 235–8. Literature, not written with ethics teaching in mind, is said to contrast with 'ethics cases', written by ethicists, who may or may not have a philosophical background and produce cases primarily as thought experiments. Often such cases are not value free; the use of the passive voice, dehumanising language and metaphors can subtly communicate a particular bias. Cf. discussions by Chambers TS (1994) The bioethicist as author: the medical ethics case as rhetorical device. *Literature and Medicine.* **13**: 60–78; (1996) From the ethicist's point of view: the literary nature of ethical inquiry. *Hastings Center Report.* **26 (1)**: 25–32; and (1999) *The Fiction of Bioethics: cases as literary texts.* Routledge, New York. Of course, the humanities can be mined in ways that inject biases into arguments. For concerns of humanities becoming the handmaiden of bioethics, Friedman LD (2002) The precarious position of the medical humanities in the medical school curriculum. *Academic Medicine.* **77**: 320–2. Friedman sees bioethics as taught to physicians as relying on principles and rules that have 'tilted bioethics more toward scientific methods of reasoning rather than humanistic interpretation of data.' Relevant, too, in raising questions about the agenda of professional ethicists, is that, working as experts in institutions, institutional legitimacy can become more of an issue than being part of public debate: Koch T (2003) Absent virtues: the poacher becomes gamekeeper. *Journal of Medical Ethics.* **29**: 337–42.

9   Quote taken from Williams' essay 'The Practice' reprinted in Reynolds R and Stone J (eds) (1991) *On Doctoring: stories, poems, essays.* Simon & Schuster, New York, p. 73. It seems appropriate to also note the views of one commentator, F Neelon, who disagrees with those who feel that the 'arts' function is merely a recreational way to divert or refresh the doctor after the toil and burdens of the medical day. Neelon believes the doctor's job is always 'an act of creative interpreting. It is analogous in detail to the reader's job of understanding the written or spoken word. The more we attune ourselves

to the "hearing" that forms the basis of careful reading ... the better we prepare ourselves for the doctor's great and fearsome task: listening to the patient's story and trying to make sense ... out of it.' (Neelon F quoted in Palmer J 'An Introduction to the Arts-for-Health Movement or How the Arts Sneaked In on the Medical Model'. www.community arts.net/readingroom/archive/intro-health.php [accessed July 2004].)

10   For such issues as medical education and the phrase moral order: Wear D and Bickel J (2000) *Educating for Professionalism: creating a culture of humanism in medical education.* University of Iowa Press, Iowa City. The qualities required to be a good physician have exercised much public thinking in recent years. It was, for instance, a specific theme in an issue of the *British Medical Journal*, 2002; **325** (28 September).

11   The programme received substantial government funding. EFPO Working Paper #1 (December 1992). For accounts: Demand-Side Medical Education: educating future physicians of Ontario; Neufeld VR, Maudsley RM, Pickering RJ *et al.* (1998) Educating future physicians for Ontario. *Academic Medicine.* **73**: 1133–48; Maudsley RF, Wilson DR, Neufeld VR *et al.* (2000) Educating future physicians for Ontario: Phase II. *Academic Medicine.* **75**: 113–26. The EFPO working papers are typescripts available through Associated Medical Services, Toronto, Ontario.

12   Listed in published articles, no. 11. In fact, the scientist-scholar role arose largely from input from medical faculty, and the role as person from medical student groups.

13   At Queen's University, see www.meds.queensu.ca/medicine/pbl/pblhome4.htm (accessed July 2004). Interpreting comments from focus groups, etc. into specific roles was not easy as evident from the reports of the working groups, where, for instance, the term 'humanist' appears, though it did not reach the final list, nor did 'healer' though that reflects many sentiments expressed. See EFPO unpublished Working Papers, 1992–93. At another medical school, at the University of Western Ontario, it has been made clear that the EFPO roles are very much part of the central philosophy of patient-centred care in a revised MD curriculum. Much has been written on this. For instance, Freeman TR (2000) UWO Family Medicine at the Millennium. www.familymedicineuwo.ca/about/article_0600.shtml (accessed July 2004).

14   As is clear from all the original reports (EFPO Working Paper Series 1–20), classifying diverse views into specific categories was open to interpretation, thus allowing a certain amount of relabelling.

15   It is appropriate to note that issues of quality of care are widely discussed in the literature, often with nuanced meanings, but with little consensus on how to measure it or its relations to professionalism. (See papers from a recent symposium on quality care, but which fail to notice professional values: Symposium on quality healthcare (2003) *Perspectives in Biology and Medicine.* **46**: 1–79.)

16   The roles are listed as 'medical expert/clinical decision maker, communicator, collaborator, manager, health advocate, scholar and professional'. See *Skills for the New Millennium.* Report of the Societal Needs Working Group, listed under publications on www. rcpsc.medical.org/publications/index.php accessed July 2004.

17   For information on the Royal College of Physicians and Surgeons of Canada, see www. rcpsc.medical.org (accessed March 2003).

18   This becomes clear in various chapters; see also Kenny NP and Mann KV (2001) See one, do one, teach one: role models and the CanMEDS competencies. *Annals of the Royal College of Physicians and Surgeons of Canada.* **34**: 435–9.

19   For the UK and US, Martin J, Lloyd M and Singh S (2002) Professional attitudes: can they be taught and assessed in medical education? *Clinical Medicine Journal of the Royal College of Physicians of London.* **2**: 217–23. Also for the UK, Irvine D (2001) Doctors in the UK: their new professionalism and its regulatory framework. *Lancet.* **358**: 1807–10.

20   The subject of a formal social contract between medicine and society has been a frequent topic of discussion from the 1980s onward. See, for example, Murray TJ (1995) Medical education and society. *Canadian Medical Association Journal.* **153**: 1443–6.

21   Cf. Ludmerer KM (1999) *Time to Heal: American medical education from the turn of the century to the era of managed care.* Oxford University Press, Oxford, pp. 304–5.

22   For concerns about lack of humanistic qualities of physicians, see Neufeld VR (1998) Physician as humanist: still an educational challenge. *Canadian Medical Association Journal.* **159**: 787–8. Multiculturalism became a critical issue in the last decades of the

twentieth century; a particular issue is tendencies to ignore or dismiss as irrational or unscientific many lay beliefs. Although it is true that they may not fit scientific concepts, the humanities help to show that, given basic premises, they can be very much based on rational thinking. The extent to which lay health practices can be described as rational has often been discussed. For one introductory discussion on a contentious area, Hufford DJ (1993) Epistemologies in religious healing. *Journal of Medicine and Philosophy.* **18**: 175–94. Hufford argues that 'attention to actual beliefs of individuals often reveals them to be rationally ordered and empirically founded.'

23 Controlled studies, as yet unpublished, have been reported by T Greenhalgh at a conference, 'The Healing Continuum: medical humanities and the good doctor', held under the auspices of New York University Postgraduate Medical School, 17–18 October 2003.

24 For one discussion on humanities in relation to humane behaviour: McManus IC (1995) Humanity and the humanities. *Lancet.* **346**: 1143–5.

25 Quoted from ibid. (Keynes G (1981) *The Gates of Memory.* Clarendon Press, Oxford.)

26 As one 2002 example: 'It may sound a little fanciful, but for me it is not an overstatement to say, that on the medical humanities [MA] course I found my 'spiritual home' in medicine. Prior to that and despite having done the membership [of the Royal College of Physicians of London] and a diploma in palliative medicine, both of which did have elements of what I was looking for, I have always felt that my medical studies omitted large chunks of things that I intuitively knew to be important. The MA course filled all the gaps and introduced me to many other people who thought the same way, which was a wonderfully validating experience.' Quoted from website October 2002, now revised (July 2004) at: www.healthscience.swan.ac.uk/Courses/Postgraduate/XMA_ Medical_ Humanities.asp. Such testimonials serve as a reminder that the long history of formal medical history courses has left a legacy of physicians who testify that history offers a way to reflect on their medical practice and, thereby, make them better doctors. Likewise there is the support of medical humanities of senior practitioners who have become well known for superior scientific or clinical work. For instance, Baum M (2002) Teaching the humanities to medical students. *Clinical Medicine Journal of the Royal College of Physicians of London.* **2**: 246–9.

27 Osler W (1919) *The Old Humanities and the New Science.* Houghton Mifflin, Boston, p. 26 for quote.

28 Downie RS (ed) (1994) *The Healing Arts: an Oxford illustrated anthology.* Oxford University Press, Oxford, p. 1.

29 The quote about changing cultures is about medical education in the US, but it has relevance elsewhere. Ludmerer KM and Fox RC (2001) Caring and medical education. In: LE Cluff and RB Binstock (eds) *The Lost Art of Caring: a challenge to health professionals, families, communities, and society.* Johns Hopkins University Press, Baltimore, pp. 125–36.

30 The issue of uncertainty is often raised in medical discussions. For an informative discussion, Fox R (1988) 'The evolution of medical uncertainty'. In her *Essays in Medical Sociology: journeys into the field.* Transaction Books, New Brunswick, pp. 533–71.

31 I am grateful to Rebecca King for her observations and permission to quote from her essay.

32 Weatherall D (1995) *Science and the Quiet Art: the role of medical research in health care.* Norton, London, p. 327.

33 Gabe J, Kelleher D and Williams G (eds) (1994) *Challenging Medicine.* Routledge, New York.

34 For direct and indirect impacts on healthcare, Morris DB (1998) *Illness and Culture in the Postmodern Age.* University of California Press, Berkeley.

35 Anonymous student assignment (1998).

36 As an illustration, experience has shown that Michael LaCombe's short story 'Playing God' (*see* Chapter 2) always elicits controversy. Academic contributions to 'literature and medicine' are now substantial. Its role for physicians can be usefully explored in Coles R (1989) *The Call of Stories: teaching and the moral imagination.* Houghton Mifflin, Boston.

37 Medical humanities resources at NYU School of Medicine: www.endeavor.med. nyu.edu/lit-med/medhum.html (accessed July 2004).

38   For illustration of medical interest in the classics: Salinsky J (2002) *Medicine and Literature: the doctor's companion to the classics.* Radcliffe Medical Press, Oxford. The discipline 'literature and medicine' explores not only the 'messages' about, for instance, patients' needs, but also the contributions of physicians and medicine to literature.

39   LaCombe M (ed) (1995) *On Being a Doctor.* American College of Physicians, Philadelphia; and LaCombe M (ed) (2000) *On Being a Doctor 2. Voices of Physicians and Patients.* American College of Physicians, Philadelphia. Other collections or anthologies are cited throughout the volume.

40   Selzer (1992) makes this clear in his memoirs, *Down from Troy: a doctor comes of age.* William Morrow, New York.

41   It is relevant that patients are not passive sponges and that they interpret information in various ways. See Davin S (2003) Healthy viewing: the reception of medical narratives. *Sociology of Health and Illness.* **25**: 662–79.

42   A key resource is Dans PE (2000) *Doctors in the Movies. Boil the Water and Just Say Aah.* Medi-Ed Press, Bloomington. Noteworthy, too, is Shortland M (1989) *Medicine and Film: a checklist, survey and research resource.* Wellcome Unit for the History of Medicine (Research Publications Number IX), Oxford. Amidst a now substantial journal literature, see 'Special Section on History of Science in Film', *Isis* (1993); **84**: 750–74.

     We stress that references to movies in this volume are not concerned with their quality, whether they be art or 'B' movies, but with their role in reflecting and reinforcing trends that shape popular attitudes. Our premise is that commercial films are an influential medium within society, particularly those films produced to appeal to a wide audience. Inherent in popular appeal is a crucial two-way communication between audience and director. Although popular films can have iconoclastic messages and themes, directors and producers, in striving for commercial success, are often in line with the experiences and ideals of the target audience.

     Negative or ambivalent images of physicians in movies, mostly 1960s and later, reinforce negative experiences increasingly spotlighted by malpractice cases; this helps to stereotype physicians and thereby reinforce challenges to the profession.

43   Pope R (1991) *Illness & Healing: images of cancer.* Lancelot Press, Hantsport. For recent article on Kahlo with bibliography, Gamble JG (2002) Frida Kahlo: her art and her orthopedics. *The Pharos.* **65 (3)**: 5–12. Kahlo became better known in the English-speaking world with the movie *Frida* (2002).

44   For the book: Ensler E (1998) *The Vagina Monologues.* Random House, New York.

45   Konner M (1987) *Becoming a Doctor: a journey of initiation in medical school.* Elizabeth Sifton, New York, p. xi.

46   Medical autobiography can be viewed as a distinct genre open to various interpretations. Cf. Pollack D (1996) Training tales: US medical autobiography. *Cultural Anthropology.* **11**: 339–61. Pollack notes that it is a relatively recent genre and differs from celebratory autobiography so common within medicine. He also comments, 'Physician training later tends to be critical of medicine, of its depersonalized, institutionalized, mechanized, bureaucratized nature.'

47   Klass P (1992) Writing is my best defense. *Journal of the American Medical Association.* **268**: 1191. Klass's *A Not Entirely Benign Procedure* was published by Putnam, New York. Other well-known books (overlapping with interning) up to the 1980s that have led to much more recent writing include: Doctor X (1965) *Intern.* Harper and Row, New York; Shem S (1978) *The House of God.* Marek, New York; LeBaron C (1981) *Gentle Vengeance.* Marek, New York; and Reilly P (1987) *To Do No Harm.* Auburn House, Dover.

48   Davies R (1994) *The Cunning Man.* McClelland and Stewart, Toronto.

49   Winckler M (2000) *The Case of Dr Sachs.* Seven Stories Press, New York (English edition), p. 112. Originally published in French, 1997.

Part 1
Foundation roles

CHAPTER 2

Doctors: how professional are they seen to be?

What is professionalism? Diverse views

> In a society constituted as are our modern states, the interests of the social order will be served best when the number of men entering a given profession reaches and does not exceed a certain ratio ... When ... six or eight ill-trained physicians undertake to gain a living in a town which can support only two, the whole plan of professional conduct is lowered in the struggle which ensues, each man becomes intent on his own practice, public health and sanitation are neglected and the ideals and standards of the profession tend to demoralization. (Abraham Flexner, 1910)[1]

Abraham Flexner's observations, published in his critical and influential 1910 report on American medical education, is just one indication that public concerns about professional matters within medicine have been around for a long time. Nevertheless, it may surprise many people that physicians in the 1990s openly debated whether professionalism should be taught *formally* in medical schools, rather than relying on time-honoured physician role models.[2] This, however, was a clear response to rising concerns expressed, within and outside the medical profession, about professional standards. 'Physicians' professionalism and humanism', it was said in 2002, 'have become central foci of the efforts of medical educators as the public, various accrediting and licensing agencies, and the profession itself have expressed concerns about the apparent erosion of physicians' competency in these aspects of the art of, rather than the science of, medicine.'[3]

This chapter looks at lay images of and attitudes toward doctors. At issue is the nature, extent and impact of the images on public perceptions of professionalism. The chapter, lengthier than others, serves to set the scene for later discussions on specific public expectations of physicians. It should become clear that public questioning of physicians has now become so commonplace that even those patients who have great trust and confidence in their physicians are likely to be more discerning in their assessments than their predecessors. One conclusion we come to in this book is that individual physicians must now *earn* respect, whereas in the past respect could just as likely be acquired by riding, as it were, on the coat-tails of the profession.[4]

Exactly what does it mean to be a professional? Like countless simple questions this one defies a simple answer, partly because it depends on who is asked. Some might say, as can be heard among physicians, that it means to be licensed and to follow a code of ethics. Another common sentiment in the early 2000s is that a professional is a highly skilled 'knowledge worker' (i.e. merely a provider of expert services). And, with many occupations claiming to be a profession in recent years, a Scott Adam's Dilbert cartoon script offered inimitable perspective by suggesting that taking more than six minutes for lunch is unprofessional.[5]

More nuanced answers to questions about professionalism come from sociologists who study the characteristics that define a profession. Depending on their particular perspectives and theories, they emphasise some or all of the following:

1   agreement on the standards of practice and codes of ethics
2   codification of knowledge through specialised education and core curricula
3   self-regulation and social closure through limiting the number of practitioners
4   generally strict alignment with the scientific paradigm
5   constant efforts to improve on the status quo
6   support from strategic elites such as the state and powerful pressure groups.[6]

Defining a profession in this way reflects the analytical approach of an academic discipline. In contrast, the eyes of the beholder, the layperson or patient, while consciously or unconsciously accepting the characteristics just mentioned, commonly views the professionalism of his or her own doctor in the light of their own experiences and perceptions. These can vary widely. They may depend, for instance, on whether the doctor is empathetic or is *seemingly* knowledgeable of medical developments. This chapter notices some general factors – hospitals and their practitioners, doctors' offices, gender stereotyping, nostalgia for the country doctor, and a patient's particular circumstances – that have had, and continue to have, an impact on how the beholder sees physicians and perceives their professionalism.

Changing images, perceptions and expectations

> The doctor tapped his desk thoughtfully for a moment, then suddenly his face lit up with some brilliant thought and he wrote out orders for five more examinations ... I didn't like the contented smile with which he handed them to me. I went out felicitating myself on having cleverly side-stepped the stomach test, but a few hours later I discovered the cause of his merriment, for I walked right into another, much worse – a cystoscopic examination – where they insert something that feels like a piece of rusty barbed wire into the bladder and up through the ureter into the kidney. Affixed to the inner end of this ingenious apparatus – which has an opening through the center – there is a tiny electric light bulb, by means of which they get a view of the interior furnishings. To facilitate this they dilate the parts by pumping in air, soda, transparent acids and suchlike pain-producing inventions. ('The Cystoscopic Trap', 1930)[7]

Hospital settings

Henry Harper, the author of the above remarks, continued by describing the extreme unpleasantness of 'probing, twisting, pumping and expanding the inside membraneous walls of the kidney' for which 'no printable language can do it justice.' Finally, he remarks that 'the only near-humorous feature that I discovered in the whole procedure was the remark of one of the examining physicians, that he didn't think it would hurt – much.'

Harper's cystocopic experience was not his only unhappy and tortuous experience with kidney disease at the Mayo Clinic, which, in the 1930s, was one of the most prestigious centres for the new 'scientific' medicine anywhere. It is revealing that the preface to Harper's book – written in a self-congratulatory tone by a physician who could hardly have read between the lines – noted that 'Mr Harper enters only one complaint against a member of my profession, and that a justifiable one: his account of the first post-operative dressing should be told to every young medical student as a warning and a threat for them to avoid such a brutal performance.'

Whether or not Harper – one of relatively few patients publishing their experiences in the first half of the twentieth century – whitewashed concerns he had about professional behaviour is unknown. He was writing during what has been called the 'Golden Age of Medicine', a time lasting until at least the 1950s, when the social standing of physicians was in the ascendant.[8] This owed much to the growth of confidence in science-based medicine and positive media coverage of medical heroes backed by improved or new diagnostic tools such as laboratory tests, striking developments in surgical and medical therapies, and the consequent expansion of hospital medicine. Relatively few voices – satire apart – openly questioned the prestige and authority of physicians, even after the exposés of questionable morals of doctors in the renowned novels *Arrowsmith* and *The Citadel* in the 1920s and '30s (*see* Chapter 5).

Although the growth of scientific medicine brought concerns that the patient was being treated less personally and humanely, a new patient era, as it can be called, only emerged after the 1960s or so.[9] Individuals with questioning, often outspoken, voices made it increasingly clear that they wished to be involved in decision making about their health and treatment. One such person was Rachel Carson, author of the acclaimed *Silent Spring* (1962), who contributed much to the changing social values of the time, at least with regard to the environment. From 1960 until her death from breast cancer in 1964, her correspondence with Dr George Crile at the renowned Cleveland Clinic is insightful at a time when breast cancer was not an experience openly shared among women, and when the patient's 'right' to question anything about the management of the disease had not yet become commonly accepted.[10] After a radical mastectomy, Carson was particularly frustrated by the realisation that she had not been told the truth about her disease; she had been led to believe it was a 'condition bordering on malignancy'.[11]

Carson was able to stand outside the immediacy of her illness and her tortuous hospital experiences; in this she was aided by Crile, even though he was in Cleveland and not Washington where Carson lived. She found in him a 'mind [that] combines everything I wanted.' 'It would be hard,' she wrote to him, 'to express fully the feeling of relief I have now that the direction of treatment is in your hands ... I appreciate, too, you having enough respect for my mentality and emotional stability to discuss all this frankly with me. I have a great deal more peace of mind when I know the facts, even though I might wish they were different.'[12] She also offered pithy comments about Washington physicians, and made it clear that she did not wish to be referred to particular practitioners on the basis of professional associations and courtesies. Crile's relationship with Carson was one signal that, in the future, individual physicians would have to forge new types of relationships with patients.

In 'Graveyard Shift', poet Anne Caston writes emotively of delivering babies wrapped in blue blankets to the cold crypts, lying in refrigerated drawers in the morgue upstairs. The grim scene gives way to the dim-lit night nursery with croup tents 'like chilly amniotic sacs'. The nurses, the poet notices, have to be prepared for a fire or tornado – some unforeseen catastrophe; they wear aprons with six pockets for carrying the babies if necessary.[13]

Caston is one of a long line of poets who have added some of the most evocative scenes of hospital life to those of patients like Harper and Carson, and to a kaleidoscope of novels, short stories, visual art, movies and media reports.[14] In general, these underscore that the twentieth-century hospital became a key part – more significant than the physician's surgery (office in North America) – of the public image of medicine. Images abound of non-stop theatre with changing scenes of patient's foreboding and fear, surrealism, horror, hope amid birth, pain and death, and community pride that often centre around physician power and authority. What is problematic for physicians, indeed for healthcare as a whole, is that negative depictions have come to overshadow positive ones (*see also* Box 2.1).[15]

Box 2.1 Hospitals: places of medical power and uncertainty

A long-standing societal fear that hospitals are places to die still colours the attitudes of many people. Moreover, hospitals have become increasingly intimidating as their complexity and technology has increased.

The complex story of hospitals extends back to the Middle Ages and earlier, but the expression 'hospital medicine' only arose – in the sense of it being a specialty – in the early decades of the twentieth century. Even so, the role of hospitals as a fountain-head of medicine, rather than solely a place to care for and treat the sick, had emerged earlier. During the eighteenth century, for instance, bringing patients together with similar conditions meant they became 'resources' for physicians and students to study 'diseases'.

Many hospitals became centres of medical education and research, and thereby contributed significantly to the development of the then relatively new clinico-pathological approach to diagnosis. The growth of the authority of regular medicine in the twentieth century owes much to the expansion of hospitals, their role as repositories of complex diagnostic technology and therapeutic devices, and in fostering specialism in medical practice that has done so much to shape healthcare. As physicians and nurses developed new roles in hospitals and as physiotherapists, X-ray technicians, dietitians and medical social workers joined them there was a closer locking together of the 'modern' physician, medical education and the hospital than ever before. Medical historian Charles Rosenberg has said (1987) in his book, *The Care of Strangers* (Basic Books, New York, p. 3), that by 1920 the hospital, as an institution, had become 'medicalized', while the medical profession had become 'hospitalized'.

Negative happenings and images

Among the negative images, movies are the most conspicuous in spotlighting, if not stereotyping, the worst side of hospitals and medical professionalism.[16] The positive scenes common during the pre-1950s, depicted by, for example, the high ideals and devotion of Drs Kildare and Gillespie (15 movies, 1937–1947), were slowly overwhelmed from the 1960s onward by a growing number of questionable depictions of physicians – mostly of psychiatrists, but also ranging from ophthalmologists to obstetricians.[17] Indeed, positive images, at least in the public's mind, serve only to highlight the greater number of negative depictions in recent times. One such positive image is of the physician Patch Adams in the 1998 movie of the same name. Adams challenges the conservatism of the medical establishment as he enhances patient care through promoting laughter.[18] While the trend away from positive movie depictions owed something to the ending of the censorship of critical depictions of the medical profession, it paralleled, and almost certainly reflected, other public voices questioning physician behaviour as well as the diminished political influence of such institutions as the American Medical Association.[19]

Although physicians have long been the butt of satirists and caricaturists, the tone changed from the 1960s onward. It shifted away from spotlighting pomposity and borderline behaviour, especially with women patients, toward much more emphasis on the abuse of power and authority over patients.[20] One sign of this questioning of professionalism is the theme of 'playing God' that depicts physicians who ignore patients and who abuse the power society accords them. Playing God scenarios, conspicuous in both novels and movies, are far removed from, say, the values that the public associate with the humaneness of the ideal physician or perceptions of archetype physicians such as Hippocrates; moreover, the theme does not allow the layperson insights into the real dilemmas facing physicians that lead to 'God-like' decisions taken in what are felt to be the best interests of a patient.[21] The dust jacket of Stanley Winchester's 1967 novel, *The Practice*, stated that it was 'a different novel of the world of medicine', and that if it raises doubts of the divine status sometimes accorded men of medicine, 'it also points to the undeniable corollary that gods do not practice medicine, men do.'[22] If there was some pulling of punches within the novel – for instance, in the statement that doctors were 'only *one* rank below God' because 'they know so much about your body'[23] – the ranking was raised some years later when a plastic surgeon, short on moral values in the movie *Without Malice* (2000), remarked: 'Unlike God, I *don't* make mistakes.' In fact, a patient in 1993, when describing his life with adrenoleukodystrophy (ALS) and relationships with physicians, had already awarded a higher accolade: 'It's been said that the primary difference between doctors and God is that God doesn't think he's a doctor.'[24]

Some further examples from popular films in the 1990s illustrate the pervasiveness of the physician as God theme. With some exceptions, when moral principles are reawakened or drug addiction overcome as in *Playing God* (1997), most such physicians met their just desserts.[25] There was, for example, surgeon Jedd Hill (in *Malice*, 1993) whose 'indulgence in the God complex' was even self-evident to medical colleagues. Most memorable, perhaps, is Dr Lawrence Myrick in *Extreme Measures* (1996), based on a medical thriller by physician Michael Palmer. As a renowned neurosurgeon/researcher on the brink of restoring transected spinal cords, Myrick recognises that, at the age of 68, his time is 'running out'. He shifts to experimenting on humans – homeless street people without their consent – to find the 'medicine no one has ever dreamed of'. These men have 'no family, nothing, no future,' says Myrick. 'They are not victims; they are heroes. Because of them, millions will walk again.' Myrick's protagonist, a young physician with ethical ideals, responds: 'Maybe they are heroes, but they didn't choose to be. You chose for them ... You can't do that, because you are a doctor and you took an oath. You're not God.'

Sometimes, the notion of the physician as God is portrayed as much by plot and atmosphere as by words. In the movie *Flatliners* (1990), a group of medical students, in an extra-curricula activity, investigate near-death experiences. After a student's heart is stopped and resuscitated before brain death, he or she shares their experiences with the group. 'Messages' from the movie, with its interior scenes conjuring gothic churches, raise questions not only about religion versus science, but also how far medical science and physicians should go in controlling life and death (*see also* Chapter 5 on the physician as scientist).[26]

Screen figures such as Hill and Myrick, along with countless flawed doctors who appear in medical thrillers – the latter commonly use hospital settings for unethical research, immoral business practices and the like (*see* Box 2.2) – hardly ease anyone's innate fears of hospitals (or of physicians). Yet perhaps even more alarming are the movies that highlight grossly ineffective administrations, of which physicians may or may not be a part. Although embroidered, they commonly resonate with anecdotal experiences and with negative media reports. The biting British satire *Britannia Hospital* (1983) reveals surly workers, incompetent administration and Frankenstein-type research; its opening scene is of an elderly cardiac patient being wheeled into the Emergency Department only to be attended (rather, *not* attended) by a staff hurrying to leave because their shift had ended. And *Article 99* (1992) follows the young and idealistic Dr Peter Morgan, who, after joining the staff of a Veteran's Administration Hospital, finds himself plunged into a medical nightmare. Doctors battle with corrupt administration and bureaucratic red tape by stealing pacemakers, hijacking supplies and scheduling unauthorised operations.

Reinforcing negative movie images are books that expose medical education and hospitals. Samuel Shem's irreverent 1978 novel, *The House of God*, has been especially influential with its astonishingly successful sales of more than two million copies in over 20 languages.[27] While innumerable physicians dismiss the book as sophomoric and, by 2000 or so, outdated, the overall message for lay readers is that the medical internships of young physicians undermine humane relationships with patients; John Updike said that the book 'does for medical training what Catch-22 did for military life – display it as a farce, a mêlée of blunderers labouring to murky purpose under corrupt and platitudinous superiors.'[28] Shem himself commented publicly (2003): 'In 1973 ... we were told to treat our patients in ways we didn't think were humane. We ran smack into the conflict between the received wisdom of the medical system and the call of the human heart.'[29] Shem's later book, *Mount Misery* (1997) – the experiences of a first-year psychiatry resident – provides an equally unappetising picture of medicine.[30] Other physicians concerned over God-like roles offer suggestions on how humanity and idealism might survive the 'gruelling path to technical competency'.[31]

Box 2.2   The medical thriller

> Medical thrillers like other thrillers are intended as entertainment, but if well-researched, they can do a lot more than just give readers delicious shivers. By exploring and dramatizing important issues in medicine, they can enlighten the public and enable them to think intelligently about what is vital to them. (*Quoted by Barbara Loe Fisher writing about Michael Palmer's FATAL on the website of New Yorkers for Vaccination, Information and Choice*)

> Medical thriller plots by Robin Cook stir darkly in the back of your mind. Organs harvested from innocent patients in quiet little clinics by diabolical, megalomaniac doctors for transplant into mafia dons. (*Amy Hauslohner in ruminating on the question: Are you an organ donor?*)

Hundreds of medical thrillers have been published in recent years, and aficionados can attend courses on 'How to Write a Medical Thriller'.* This loose genre covers much criminal and immoral behaviour set in medical, invariably hospital, settings; plots range from the intricacies and successes of forensic pathologists/medical examiners to the terrors, or potential terrors, of epidemic infectious diseases.

One aspect of the success of medical thrillers is that they offer credible medical detail, especially when written by physicians. Robin Cook, for instance, is considered to be a key founder of the modern medical thriller genre with his first novel *Coma* (1977). He is known for his precise medical information in 23 thrillers. Critics have commented that Cook falls short on characterisation, as do other thriller writers; however, this can be overlooked by readers who revel more in the medical settings for villains and good guys, and who relish the fall of powerful physicians undone by their crimes.

Whatever the quality of the writing, thrillers commonly send out alarms about many aspects of medicine, especially with regard to its technology and to physician immorality. Countless ethical considerations are spotlighted, not infrequently in the context of medical technology and artificial reproduction, genetic engineering and obstetrics. Hospitals and obstetrics/gynaecology, in fact, are a fairly common setting for emotive plots. Paul Carlson's *The Scalpel* (1997), for example, is set in Dublin's Central Maternity Hospital where a baby is kidnapped and a drug-addicted obstetrician turns to murder to hide his own condition of AIDS. In dealing with contemporary medical issues, *The Scalpel* might well be seen as updating an early novel by another physician Michael Crichton: *A Case of Need* (1968), which centres around illegal abortions. There is, too, physician David Hellerstein's *Stone Babies* that can be purchased on the Internet through Electron Press; it is said to 'leave the reader with a healthy skepticism of the goings-on at prestigious hospitals, and fully educated on the inequity of medical care [in the US].'

Amid the entertainment, the fast pace, the mystery and the flawed characters, there is much to ponder over the public image of medicine and the current calls for greater levels of professionalism. Sometimes this is expressed explicitly. At the end of his novel *Vector*, Robin Cook challenges the medical profession with his view that the 'profession's responsibility with regard to bioterrorism goes beyond detecting an episode and treating its victims. The medical profession has an ethical duty to continue to institutionalize the opprobrium currently associated with the bioweapons.'

*For a comprehensive list, including physician authors: www.Medical-Thriller.com

Function and efficiency

> Everyone's distracted.
> It's clear we all hate hospitals,
> detest the pretense of order,
> abhor the charts and schedules,
> the urgent, joyless footsteps of nurses.[32]

> Here everything is white and clean
> as driftwood. Pain is localized
> and suffering, strictly routine,
> goes on behind a modest screen.[33]

One of the noticeable features of hospitals in the twentieth century is the language of functionalism, of maximum administrative efficiency. In impacting on health-care in a number of ways, many believe that it undermined humane care by physicians and others. One interesting way to reflect on this – a byway of medical humanities – is to look at hospital buildings as if they are museum artefacts. By so doing, such questions arise as to what extent hospital designs are shaped by medical concepts, and, in turn, how design shapes atmosphere and behaviour, matters that deserve at least brief comment.

Increasingly in the twentieth century, function rather than facade became reflected in the multi-storey concrete blocks that replaced pavilion-style buildings, particularly in the US. Piling one floor on top of another (made possible with new building techniques) effected economies in space, heating, supervision, cleaning and the energies of staff.[34] The trend to taller buildings – far removed from small community hospitals – coincided, at least in the US, with the growth in the popularity of the term 'medical center', which came into prominence in the 1920s and '30s to cover new partnerships between institutions. The growth of specialism within medicine at the time is also evident with such institutions as those creating the New York Medical Center. Picture postcards published in the 1930s proudly pronounced that the Center comprised the Presbyterian Hospital, the College of Physicians and Surgeons of Columbia University, the Sloane Hospital for Women, the New York State Psychiatric Institute and Hospital, the Babies' Hospital, the Squier Urological Clinic, the Presbyterian School of Nursing, the Neurological Institute and Hospital, The Stephen V Harkness Patient Pavilion, the School of Dental and Oral Surgery, the Vanderbilt Clinic and the DeLamer Institute of Public Health.[35] While this might engender civic pride in medical progress, it also made services bewilderingly complex to patients.

A later postcard (1990s) centred on the quote: 'I would rather be kept in the efficient if cold altruism of a large hospital than expire in a gush of sympathy in a small one.'[36] In fact, this sentiment, voiced by Aneurin Bevan, a political pioneer of the British National Health Service (commenced 1948), was used on the card with heavy irony to pinpoint late twentieth-century patients' disquiet with the functionalism of large hospitals, disquiet that sometimes focused on physicians as key personnel. Even though patients' voices, by the 1990s, had already led to Patients' Bills of Rights and hospital codes of ethics, questions persisted whether most modern hospitals offer true healing environments (cf. 'Places of healing' in Chapter 4).[37]

The waiting room, surgery (office) and attire – symbols of authority

> While I waited I subjected the doctor to a preliminary semiotic scrutiny. Sitting in his office I read his signs. The diplomas I took for granted: What interested me was the fact that the room was furnished with taste. There were well-made, well-filled bookcases, an antique desk and chairs, a reasonable Oriental rug on the floor.

The writer, Anatole Broyard, continues by noting photographs of three healthy-looking and happy children in a prosperous setting of lawn, flowers and trees, and on a sailboat. The conclusion was that, from the evidence, 'their father knew how to live – and, by extension, how to look after the lives of others. His magic seemed good.'[38]

Although hospitals play a key role in the public image of medicine and its professionalism, other considerations include waiting rooms, physicians' surgeries (offices in North America), and attire that runs from open-neck shirts to white coats. These receive relatively little attention from the medical profession, even though individuals may view them as indicators of a practitioner's respect for patients and for professionalism.

Nowadays, waiting rooms and physicians' surgeries, ranging widely between utilitarian rooms in a shopping centre to being part of a 'fancy' clinic, can affect patients in different ways. Waiting rooms, in particular, witness many episodes of human drama unseen by doctors. Insights are thereby lost. The following rather amusing scene in Margaret Lawrence's *The Stone Angel* (1964) captures curiosity, nervousness and tension between Hagar Shipley, a defiant 90-year-old, and her daughter-in-law Doris.

> 'Come and sit down, Mother.' It's Doris's voice, hissing at me, and I see now that I am in the doctor's waiting-room, standing here gawking at a picture of a river in spring. Have I been mumbling aloud? I can't for the life of me say. The room is full of curious eyes. Nervously, I plunge back to the chair.
>
> 'I only wanted to have a look. Just two pictures he's got – fancy that. You'd think a man in his position could afford to do a little better, wouldn't you?'
>
> 'Sh – sh –' Doris looks embarrassed, and I wonder if my voice has been louder than I realized. 'This is the way he wants it, Mother. Both

those pictures cost plenty, you can bank on that. People don't hang up dozens any more.'

She thinks she knows everything there is to know, that woman. 'Did I say dozens? Did I? I only said two wasn't many, that's all.'

'Okay, okay,' she whispers. 'People are listening, Mother.'

People are always listening. I think it would be best if one paid no heed. But I can't blame Doris. I've said the very same thing to Bram. *Hush. Hush. Don't you know everyone can hear? ...*

Finally I'm called ...[39]

Returning to Broyard's observations about a doctor's office quoted above, he goes on to say that he was shattered to find that he had been waiting in the wrong office! It turns out that the 'modern and anonymous' office of the physician he did see contributed to the 'negative feeling' he had about the doctor 'from the beginning'.[40] Just how offices might impact on patients in general can be pondered from another byway of medical humanities – the photographic record and artists' renditions of waiting-rooms and offices.[41] Of course, not everyone feels comfortable in the more elegant offices or waiting-rooms as was Broyard. Others may be intimidated or uncomfortable in a handsome office with tasteful furniture that has always sent a 'message' of success and stability. A contrasting view to Broyard's is that such offices are more for the benefit of the staff and the doctors themselves. 'If I was sick, I wouldn't care if there was an aquarium or not, as long as someone would listen to my complaint, investigate the complaint, and put me on the road to wellness.'[42]

'Mid-way' offices – reflected in one physician's jest that 'a doctor's office should be decorated tastefully, but not expensively, unless he prefers a burglar over a janitor' – are perhaps those that meet most patients' comfort levels today.[43] In fact, analogous thoughts arise out of a recent study of the healing practices of the Navaho people:

In the contemporary physician's office, the process of encountering a doctor might be altered to better reflect everyday life. A waiting room can look more like a living room, even including music or television. Patients, staff and physicians can be encouraged to contribute their own artwork for display ...[44]

Another professional consideration for physicians, although nowadays seemingly dismissed by many, is attire. During the Golden Age of Medicine up to the 1950s or so, images of doctors, at least of 'city docs', often showed them in full sartorial splendour, as in morning suits (*see* Figure 2.1). The latter was virtually a professional dress, which cartoonists, by sharply contrasting with the dress of lower class patients, signalled professional authority. By the 1950s, however, the white coat had become the generally recognised dress, although exemptions existed as in Britain where most consultant physicians eschewed the white coat, and thereby maintained a hierarchical tradition over junior staff. However, white coat exemptions were spreading at the time, especially in general practice and paediatrics; increasingly, many physicians viewed the coat as an authoritarian barrier between themselves and patients, or even as a symbol of medical science rather than of patient care. Concerns about authoritarian barriers are also raised in connection with the White Coat Ceremony (a presentation of white coats to new medical students) that was rapidly taken up, particularly by US medical schools, in the 1990s. Vigorous debates have occurred over the pro and cons of the ceremony. Some see it as a way to encourage a sense of professionalism and humanism, whereas others view it more as trying to instil a sense of medical authority or to consolidate the social prestige of physicians. In fact, both views have merit, and, in part, reflect substantial differences in the ceremonies from school to school, as well as differing interpretations on the part of students.[45]

Nowadays, it is not uncommon to find physicians dressed very informally, without a white coat, while seeing patients: open-neck shirts for men practitioners, and, occasionally, shorts for women. Patients' responses are variable depending on social class and other circumstances. Some people, like Hagar Shipley, may wear their best clothes for a visit to the doctor. Physicians have to consider that the most appropriate dress is likely to be that which meets the majority of their patients' expectations and comfort. Moreover, it is always to be borne in mind that some level of formality, perhaps white coats, remains part of medicine's stereotype image.[46]

Sexual abuse/physician stereotyping

Any consideration of public views of the professionalism of physicians must recognise a particularly conspicuous change since the 1980s. This is that stories of sexual abuse of patients and of impaired physicians stand out amid a catalogue of negative images in movies, patients' 'horror' stories of medical encounters, glib media accounts of medical mistakes, and reports of criminal behaviour (even multiple murders).[47] Even if only applicable to a very small percentage of physicians, accounts of sexual transgressions – from clear-cut abuse of professional power to charges of unnecessary hysterectomies by male gynaecologists, or to a patient's suspicion that a breast examination has gone beyond strict professional guidelines – have become a pervasive dark stain on the image of professionalism.[48]

Hollywood draws on public concerns, from the rather subtle abuse in the 1992 *The Hand that Rocks the Cradle* (obstetrician Dr Mott surreptitiously removes his glove as he prepares to do a pelvic examination on a pregnant woman) to kinky behaviour with infertile women by drug-addicted gynaecologists – the identical twin brothers in *Dead Ringers* (1988). The latter movie, with its scenes of grotesque, gold surgical instruments and red theatre gowns, leaves indelible negative images in the minds of many women.[49] Notable, too, is the true story, dramatised in *I Accuse*, a 2003 Canadian movie of a physician who attempted to avoid charges of raping patients by inserting into his own arm a plastic tube full of another man's blood. This was situated such that the blood samples taken for DNA matching in 1992, 1994 and 1996 came from the foreign blood, not his own.[50]

Somewhat more subtle images perpetuate notions of male physicians as womanisers, views that are hardly dented by the medical profession's zero-tolerance policy (established by the 1990s) toward a physician's sexual abuse of patients. Movies, some consider, have devoted more time to portraying doctors and medical students as having easy access to sex (usually with nurses and technicians) than actually taking care of patients.[51] *Critical Care* (1997), for instance, has been described by one physician as 'just the kind of film that physicians should watch,

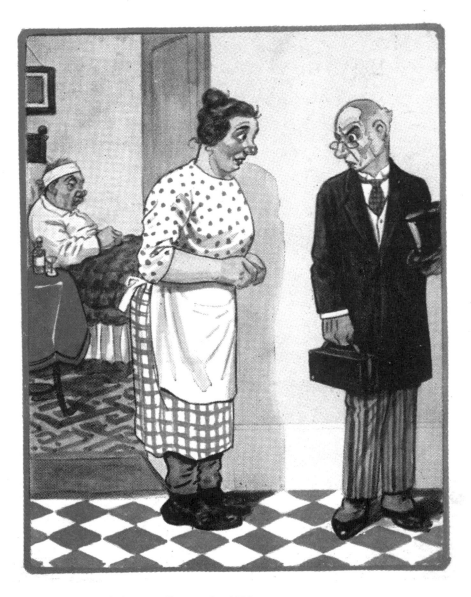

Figure 2.1 Sartorial elegance. Postcard c. 1930.

not for entertainment, but to see the extreme boundary of public attitudes.'[52] In one scene, a nurse tells Dr Ernst that she worried about him: a 'life without sleep and prodigious sex is not healthy.' Ernst himself expressed the concerns often heard about physicians, that they are only interested in 'making money, getting a new car, meeting pretty women, becoming a big-shot doctor when I should have cared about the patient, my patient.' One noteworthy reinforcement – some see it as factual – of the stereotyping appears on the opening page of the already mentioned, widely read *The House of God*: 'I and other interns handled sex. Without love, amidst the gomers and the old ones dying and the dying young, we had savaged the women of the House. From the most tender nursing school novitiate through the hard-eyed nurses of the Emergency Room, and even in pidgin Spanish, to the bangled and whistling Hispanic ones in Housekeeping and Maintenance.'[53]

Physicians are also seen as womanisers outside of their medical practices. Noteworthy is Milan Kunderer's critically acclaimed novel *The Unbearable Lightness of Being* (1984, and 1987 movie version). The principal character, a successful young surgeon, attempts to escape from the mundane world into a world of sexuality that holds no personal commitment or responsibility – one might say with clinical detachment, an issue discussed in Chapter 8. However, in a complex story of turmoil in Czechoslovakia, the philandering spirit and avoidance of commitment is constantly challenged by politics and personal relationships, just as patients constantly challenge a physician's detachment.

Although woman physicians are rarely seen to abuse patients, unflattering images abound, albeit rarely so extreme as the offhand remark, heard in the movie *A Lapse of Memory* (1992), that 'women become doctors because at heart they are either sadists or nuns.' With few exceptions, women doctors have fared badly, or are at least portrayed ambivalently, in Hollywood.[54] From the time of the movie *Coma* (1978), based on the novel of the same title by Robin Cook, they are invariably depicted with either a hard edge to their character – some can see this as part of the new feminist agenda – or emotionally vulnerable. Female psychiatrists, it seems, are most readily stereotyped as prey to unprofessional sexual affairs with patients, although sometimes with positive outcomes for the happiness of the practitioner or patient as in *Spellbound* (1945), *The Prince of Tides* (1991) and, perhaps, *Mr Jones* (1993).[55] Emotional vulnerability is further raised in *City of Angels* (1998) in which the key character, a woman cardiothoracic surgeon, is smart, and of a no-nonsense disposition until the death of one of her patients. She is also weak in communication skills, at least when one patient asks why his operation was cancelled. She told him: 'circumstances were not optimal for the procedure.' He responded that he was not a 'procedure'.

Perhaps the stereotype of a hard-edged female practitioner still owes something to assumptions of what was once necessary for pioneering women to breach all-male medical schools, and of opinions about what is still needed in certain specialty areas of medicine. Although the sense of pioneering – documented in innumerable autobiographies – had vanished by the end of the twentieth century with large numbers of women entering the profession, issues remain as is clear from Dr Frances Conley's riveting 1998 autobiography *Walking Out on the Boys*. In describing her resignation as a professor of neurosurgery at California's Stanford medical school, she exposes the worst side of academic medicine with its high proportion of prima donnas.[56]

Public responses to physician stress

No other man, unless it was Doc Hill,
Did more for people in this town than I.
And all the weak, the halt, the improvident
And those who could not pay flocked to me.
I was good-hearted, easy Doctor Meyers.
I was healthy, happy, in comfortable fortune,
Blest with a congenial mate, my children raised,
All wedded, doing well in the world.
And then one night, Minerva, the poetess,
Came to me in her trouble, crying.
I tried to help her out – she died –
They indicted me, the newspapers disgraced me,
My wife perished of a broken heart.
And pneumonia finished me.[57]

The way public attitudes can change is always an issue for physicians. Alcohol and drug abuse – not uncommonly linked to physician stress – offers a noteworthy example. This goes beyond the fickleness of public opinion as hinted at by Doctor Meyers in Edgar Lee Masters' classic *Spoon River Anthology* (1916) of voices from the graveyard.

There is no reason to think that Meyers' difficulty led him to alcohol or drugs, although alcoholic physicians are not uncommon in novels, short stories and movies. Perhaps the best known is the title character in William Carlos Williams' short story, *Old Doc Rivers* (1932). Addicted to dope and known to other physicians for making mistakes, Doc Rivers was nevertheless held in high esteem by his patients: 'they believed in him: Rivers, drunk or sober.'[58] If, today, this seems a paradox, it is because of a change in levels of public tolerance. No longer will comments be heard such as the following about a doctor, not fictional, in Newfoundland: 'by 1950 it was no secret. Dr Olds drank like a fish. "Who wouldn't?" said a knowing friend. People wondered how he bore so much without cracking. He did so because he had guts, a loving mate, a strong mother, faithful friends. *He also had a crutch*.'[59] And, earlier, another small community accepted the practice of a physician's wife in raising or lowering a flag according to whether the physician was sober and available for visits.[60] Just as telling in suggesting a level of public acceptance in the past is the alcohol-impaired physician who is incidental to the main plot of a story. An example appears in Robertson Davies' *Fifth Business* (1970) when the doctor came, rather drunk, but fairly capable and was able to reapply a dressing and give an injection.[61]

Nowadays any sign of substance abuse questions professional standards, indicative of a substantial change in public attitudes. Even the sight of medical students boisterously drinking in public bars can occasion negative public comment. This – perhaps all the public sees of the students *en masse* – is a reminder of Shem's *The House of God* in which the narrator, on vacation just after finishing the year of internship, admits to being drunk much of the time, and that 'alcohol helped in the House of God' (the hospital); he also recalls his 'best friend, Chuck, the black intern from Memphis, who was never without a pint of Jack Daniels in his black bag for those extra-bitter times when he was hurt by the gomers or the slurping house academics.'[62]

Despite awareness of doctors like Rivers and Olds, the medical profession, at a time when whistle blowing on colleagues was generally frowned upon, commonly turned a blind eye on errant colleagues until at least the 1970s and '80s. One well-known conundrum in the history of medicine surrounds the drug addiction of surgeon William Halsted (1852–1922). Best known for his radical mastectomy operation, Halsted made many other significant contributions to surgery as well as to the development of the renowned Johns Hopkins medical school and hospital. Early in his career, he became addicted to cocaine when investigating its anaesthetic properties on himself and on colleagues and students. Although weaned from cocaine, he developed lifelong dependency on daily doses of morphine. The extent to which this was known to colleagues remains debatable, but it hints at the turning of many blind eyes, something no longer sanctioned by the public.[63]

Just as turning a blind eye on physician substance abuse was no longer socially acceptable by the last decades of the twentieth century, the public raised new levels of concerns over physician stress. A particular issue voiced by many is sleep deprivation and its potential effects on the safety of practice. One poet included it along with drugs and alcohol:

> Some of them smoke marijuana
> and are alcoholics, and their moral
> turpitude is famous: who gets to see
> most sex organs in the world? Not
> poets. With the hours they keep
> they need the drugs more than anyone.[64]

Even with growing public appreciation of new stresses brought about by changes in the working environments of today's physicians – new diseases such as AIDS and SARS, new expectations and demands from patients, media exposure of mistakes, high rates of malpractice litigation and other frustrations – the public no longer accepts 'crutches' as was once the case.[65]

Nostalgia for the country doc

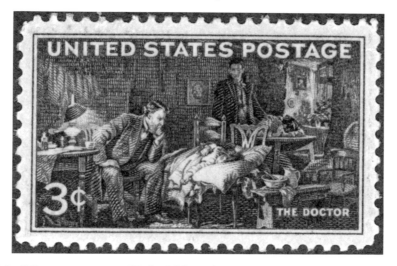

Figure 2.2   US postage stamp of Luke Fildes' *The Doctor*.

Luke Fildes' celebrated painting of a physician, watching over a child in a humble home, has become an icon medical image (*see* Figure 2.2). It became one of the most widely reproduced pictures – and the inspiration for others – during the twentieth century, especially the first half. More than a million engravings of it appeared in the United States in parlours and physicians' waiting rooms. One noteworthy aspect of the picture's story was its use by the American Medical Association as part of its campaign (1949–1952) against socialised medicine in order to suggest that the type of care depicted would be lost.[66]

'The Doctor' is but one example of many paintings that, in featuring doctor and patient, sharpen debate about physician–patient relationships. In recent decades the clinical encounter has virtually disappeared from the work of visual artists. It is suggested that, nowadays, conventional medicine is depicted as 'ambiguous and alien' while there is a 'focus on holistic notions of healing, thus avoiding bio-medicine altogether; or with a focus on the subjective experience of illness, thus ignoring the interaction between medicine and the diseased person.'[67]

Contrasting with the negative to ambivalent pictures of physicians noted so far, but in many ways highlighting them, are images of the 'good' or the 'ideal' physician. Anatole Broyard, for instance, wished for internationally known physician Oliver Sacks, with his reputation as a humanist, while Rachel Carson found her support and strength in George Crile.

A question arises whether for many people, especially older citizens, the ideal is shaped, at least in part, by images of 'old-timer' doctors who provided constant services to patients and their community. To what extent does nostalgia enter the picture? Considering this question opens a by-way of medical humanities, namely frequent reminders of the old days through, for instance, rural doctor biographies and autobiographies, museum exhibits and characters in novels.[68] Country doctors, who generally practised without the plush offices and handsome buggies or automobiles of many city physicians, and who were ready – twenty-four hours a day, seven days a week – to undertake strenuous house calls are very much part of the persistent images of caring doctors.[69]

At the time Luke Fildes' picture was becoming well known, a number of movies were also fostering the image of the caring, of the 'good', doctor. An early example is the 1909 silent film, *The Country Doctor*. In this melodrama of heroism and tragedy, the country doctor's sense of duty led him to save one child by ignoring entreaties to return to his home to look after his own sick child, who died as a consequence. And, in 1936, *The Country Doctor* (1936) – a romanticised portrayal of Canadian general practitioner Allan Dafoe who delivered the celebrated Dionne quintuplets – sent audiences 'out of the theatre to the sound of stirring music, with as good a feeling about doctors as from any movie ever made.'[70]

Such images, rose-tinted and with rough edges smoothed over, publicised ideals of commitment and service; they helped to establish universal expectations at a time when, for financial and geographical reasons, many people had little access to doctors. Yet it is noteworthy that positive country doctor images continue to be updated from time to time. In 1998, a *Life* magazine article, 'What Makes a Good Doctor? Practicing Medicine the Old Fashioned Way', described a Maine physician, who was 'inspired by the archetype of the good doctor who makes house calls with a little black bag and a great big heart. The good doctor is smart, compassionate, dedicated, thoughtful, funny and kind. He cares about all the right things – about love and honor and ethics and community. He has faith in himself, in his profession and in those he serves.'[71]

The physician in question, David Loxterkamp, had in fact already received acclaim for his book, *A Measure of My Days: the journal of a country doctor* (1997), in which he chronicles a year in his life as a rural family physician.[72] Echoing other physicians during the 1990s, Loxterkamp felt that traditional values were being diluted in medicine: 'Through my practice I have discovered what Sir William Osler, father of American medicine, once observed: "Nothing will sustain you more potently than the power to recognize in your humdrum routine, as perhaps it may be thought, the true poetry of life – the poetry of the commonplace, of the ordinary man, of the plain, toil-worn woman, with their loves and their joys, their sorrows and griefs."'[73]

The persistent image of the old country doc points up the early twenty-first century angst of the public and the medical profession, especially in North America, about how to ensure sufficient numbers of physicians practise in rural areas and hold values such as expressed by Loxterkamp. Here we just notice that, in general, the profession pays little attention to how medical humanities might contribute to the life of a rural physician; it can, for instance, sharpen the ability to observe people and their communities, even ways to 'belong', rather than merely to 'live' in, a community. A fascinating book, Gerald Pocius' *A Place to Belong*, explores in great detail how the inhabitants of one small community in Canada know every space, meadow, building as part of their sense of belonging.[74] It may well be that the sense of belonging among those living in Pocius' community differs from those elsewhere in North America and certainly other countries, but the account adds to other evocative books that directly or indirectly raise questions about doctors living in small communities; one book is the now classic *The Story of a Country Doctor: a fortunate man*, by John Berger and Jean Mohr, which follows the life of a British general practitioner at a time of major changes in medicine.[75]

Patients examine their own practitioners

The title of one of Broyard's essays, 'The Patient Examines the Doctor', is a reminder that patients' perceptions of physicians can be shaped by factors other than the general aura of hospitals, offices, attire and the 'horror' stories about physician abuse of patients, stress and burn-out that have been considered so far. Personal situations and experiences can be just as important. Here we notice four voices to illustrate just how individual circumstances of a patient can shape their attitudes toward a health professional who is unlikely to recognise the situation.

The continuation of Mrs Hagar Shipley's visit to the doctor – after her waiting-room experience quoted earlier – spotlights seemingly small and inconsequential points and discriminatory attitudes perceived by the elderly. First Mrs Shipley observed that her daughter-in-law spoke to Dr Corby as 'though she'd left me at home'.

> 'Her bowels haven't improved one bit. She's not had another gall-bladder attack, but the other evening she threw up. She's fallen a lot –'
> And so on and so on. Will she never stop? My meekness of a moment ago evaporates. She's forfeited my sympathy now, meandering

on like this. Why doesn't she let me tell him? Whose symptoms are they, anyhow?

Doctor Corby is middle-aged, and the suggestion of gray in his hair is so delicately distinguished it looks as though he's had a hairdresser do it for him on purpose. He has a sharp and worldly look behind his glasses, which have mannish frames of navy blue. Before we came, Doris maintained that on a warm day like this, I'd perspire and spoil my lilac silk, but I wore it despite her. I'm glad I did. At least it clothes me decently. I never have believed a woman should look more of a frump than nature decreed for her.

Doctor Corby turns to me, smiles falsely, as though he practiced diligently every morning before a mirror.

'Well, how are you, young lady?'

Oh, now I wish I'd worn my oldest cotton housedress, the one that's ripped under the arms, and not bothered to comb my hair at all. I wish I had the nerve to conjure up and hurl at him one of Bram's epithets.

Instead, I fix him with a glance glassy and hard as cat's-eye marbles, and say nothing. He has the grace to blush. I don't relent. I glare like an old malevolent crow, perched silent on a fence, ready to caw and startle the children when they expect it least. Oh, how I am laughing inwardly, though.

Then, swiftly, the tables turn. He bids me disrobe, holds out a stiff white gown. Then he walks out of the room. Why bother granting this vestige of privacy, when all's to be known and looked at, poked and prodded, in only a moment?

'I told you this dress was foolish,' Doris grumbles. 'It's so hard to get out of.'

Finally it's done, and I am swathed in the white canvas and resemble a perambulating pup-tent.

'I don't care for these things. My, I do look a sight, don't I?'

But laughter is only a thin cloak for my shame. Hippocrates' suave descendant returns, with his voice of careful balm.

'Fine, fine. That's fine, Mrs. Shipley. Now, if you'd just get up on the examining table. Here, let the nurse help you. There. That's just fine. Now, a deep breath –'

At last it's over, his coldly intimate touch, Doris and the nurse pretending not to look, I grunting like a constipated cow in a disgust as pure as hatred.

'I think we should have some X-rays,' he says to Doris. 'I'll make the appointments for you. Would Thursday be all right, for a start?'

'Yes, yes, of course. Which X-rays, Doctor Corby?'

'We'd be safest to do three, I think. Kidneys, of course, and gall bladder, and the stomach. I hope she'll be able to keep the barium down.'

'Barium? Barium? What's that?' my voice erupts like a burst boil.

Doctor Corby smiles. 'Only something you have to drink for this particular X-ray. It's rather like a milkshake.'

The liar. I know it'll be like poison.

Dr Corby's attitude might well be described as paternalism, or 'Doctor knows best', a patronising attitude among some physicians, a real or perceived attitude increasingly challenged since the 1960s.

A second instance where a practitioner's professional manner is interpreted in a way a health professional will commonly fail to anticipate appears in the movie *Whose Life is it Anyway* (1981), still well known for publicly raising medical ethical issues at a time of less sensitivity to them.[76] The viewer sees sculptor and patient Ken Harrison, a quadriplegic following an automobile accident, clashing time and time again with his physicians and other healthcare professionals as he demands to be allowed to die by turning off his life support.[77] In one clash Harrison challenged the professional demeanour of an occupational therapist in saying that 'Every single time that I say something even a little bit awkward, you just pretend that I haven't said anything at all. It's amazing. Why can't you relate to your patients like human beings?' When the therapist responded by telling him he was getting angry and 'I can understand your anger', Harrison explosively retorted: 'Oh Jesus, you're doing it again, just listen to yourself. I said something offensive about you and you have turned your professional cheek. If you were a human being or if you were treating me like a human being, you would have told me to screw off.'

That totally unexpected imaginings can shape a patient's attitudes – even if temporarily – toward a physician is suggested in an amusing episode in Margaret Atwood's novel, *Bodily Harm* (1982).[78] The immediate experience of a freelance magazine writer, Rennie, following breast surgery was to fall in love with the surgeon. When emerging from the anaesthesia, she found her surgeon was looking at her: 'It's all right, he said. It was malignant but I think we got it all ... Now you go to sleep, he said. I'll be back.' Rennie, however, 'fell in love with him because he was the first thing she saw after her life had been saved.' She rationalised it as being imprinted 'like a duckling, like a baby chick.' She knew about imprinting for she had once written a profile for *Owl Magazine* of a man who believed geese should be used as a safe and loyal substitute for watchdogs. 'It was best to be there yourself when the goslings came out of the eggs, he said. Then they'd follow you to the ends of the earth.' That Rennie felt she was behaving like a goose put her in a foul temper.

Atwood, through Rennie, goes on to notice changing attitudes toward doctors. They were once 'functionaries' that mothers hoped daughters would marry. However, that was the fifties, which were now *passé*. In fact, falling in love with a doctor was for 'middle-aged married women' or 'women in the soaps, women in nurse novels and in sex-and-scalpel epics with titles like *Surgery* and nurses with big tits and doctors who looked like Dr Kildare on the covers.'

The last voice illustrated here, Evan Handler's, from his *Time on Fire. My Comedy of Terror* (1996) paints a different picture from the three voices just heard in pointing up a positive patient–physician relationship as Handler lives with his experiences of myelogenous leukaemia.[79] Handler sees his current physician, 'Julia', as a 'very attractive, warm, energetic woman who is not so very much older than I am.' She can tease him about a TV sitcom he made: 'Oh, boy! Did that stink,' she says, every time I see her. Handler relates how such bantering could turn into positive support. When he said that his experiences had led him to be a miser of his time, Julie looked into his eyes and said: 'That's great. You've been through a lot. Your perspective has changed. That's a good thing. You don't know how long you're going to be around – no one knows how many years they've got – but you've learned that better than most people ever have to. You should only do what you want to be doing with those moments.' Handler continues his account to make clear that effective communication was central to his positive relationship. It is a reminder of a distinction made between an ethics of decision making and an ethics of relationships with patients. The former tends to typify hospital care where a patient's autonomy is vulnerable and needs protection; the latter, more characteristic of general practice, allows a physician to educate a patient in ways that enhances relationships.[80]

Professional responses

In bringing together many voices from medical humanities – of novelists, medical thriller writers, artists and movies – that portray physicians who are flawed, and patients who are sometimes angry, sometimes mystified by their care, it is clear, despite many positive images, that noticeable levels of bemusement, uncertainty and disquiet about the medical profession existed at the end of the twentieth century.

Given this, which is in line with many social science studies that spotlight public disquiet, it is not surprising that, increasingly by the 1990s, individual physicians and medical organisations were responding.[81] Three physicians, who in effect spoke for many, are offered as additional examples to Loxterkamp, already noted. In 1996, American physician Bernard Lown summed up the opinions of many in saying that medicine's profound crisis was much deeper than ballooning costs: 'In my view, the basic reason is that medicine has lost its way, if not its soul. An unwritten covenant between doctor and patient, hallowed over several millennia, is being broken.'[82] And, later, George Lundberg in *Severed Trust: why American medicine hasn't been fixed* considered why there was a general perception that physicians cover up, close ranks and sometimes bury their mistakes.[83]

Among individuals who have consistently raised questions and reflections in professional medical journals about physicians' values and ethical behaviour, Michael LaCombe is prominent. He is one who has continued the long history of homilies to physicians and students about medical values and patient care through the effective use of the essay and short story.[84] In a 1993 article, he offers views on professionalism that are vastly different from the analytical approach of sociologists (noted earlier), and, in fact, much nearer to the 'eye of the beholder' evaluation among patients. 'Professionalism is something everyone else seems to have more of than you yourself could ever hope for. Like the sun, it can dazzle you when it strikes you unaware, and like the sun at three in the afternoon, it can both fill you full and cast a shadow.' LaCombe continues by noting that one cannot have just a little professionalism. On the other hand, some people, prima donnas, have too much of it and so they can't really be called professional. 'Professionalism follows the laws of physics and the Heisenberg Uncertainty Principle specifically, because as soon as you point to it, professionalism is no longer there. It is not a matter of *trying*. It is a matter of *being*.'[85]

LaCombe clearly sees professionalism as far more than behaviour mandated by codes of ethics as he underscores the importance of attitudes and values, and notices that professionalism can get lost in the noise of fame, achievement, power and money. He adds: 'doctors *want* to have professionalism, but too often want it to *seem*, rather than to *be*. And with seeming as with awareness, professionalism is lost.'

'Official' responses from medical institutions to public concerns about the professionalism of physicians have come from both sides of the Atlantic; for example, alongside the already considered Educating Future Physicians of Ontario project, the American Board of Internal Medicine promoted *Project Professionalism* (commenced 1990), while the British General Medical Council has called for a 'new professionalism'.[86] The American Board has established a 'set of professional responsibilities' to reaffirm 'the fundamental and universal principles and values of medical professionalism, which remain ideals to be pursued by all physicians.' The responsibilities cover ten commitments: professional competence, honesty with patients, confidentiality, appropriate relations with patients, quality of care, access to care, just distribution of finite resources, scientific knowledge, maintaining trust by managing conflicts of interest, and professional responsibilities.[87] Underpinning these are 'elements of professionalism' – traditional values – listed as altruism, accountability, duty, excellence, honour and integrity, and respect for others.[88] These concepts of professionalism are to be 'inculcated' within training programmes.[89] In fact, just as the Royal College of Physicians and Surgeons of Canada has moved to evaluate competency to fulfil physician roles in residency training, so the accreditation Council for Graduate Medical Education in the United States will require documentation that professionalism is taught, beginning in 2007.[90]

However, the question arises, how far can one assess the impact of such charters of professionalism on trainees? Some argue that reading literature from the humanities should be part of training values, for it allows a physician or student to move away from 'abstract theorising and descriptors of what professionalism is.'[91] For example, physician Rafael Campo's autobiographical essay, 'Like a Prayer', can be used to illustrate the value of altruism. In evocative language, Campo describes how his attitude toward a 'filthy junkie' patient changed. In fact, Campo's stories, essays and poems as a whole justify close attention for their challenge to every physician to consider their own values, weaknesses and barriers to effective relationships with patients.

One Campo challenge raises issues similar to those that surround wearing a white coat, namely barriers between physician and patient. In his own practice Campo sees a particular barrier arising from the authority of 'the MD after my name, so long interposed between me and the world of the infirm, that professional appendage sheathed in protective latex, an anti-penis designed to keep me disengaged, sexless, AIDS-free and possibly straight.'[92] Psychiatrist Samuel Shem, in his novel *Mount Misery*, seemingly offers a similar sentiment, albeit less graphically: 'if we can just stop acting like doctors, then [people] stop acting like patients, and things *move*.'[93] Of course, one dilemma for doctors is that not all patients are comfortable with, indeed not ready for, what can be called the democratisation of medical authority.

The next chapters

Although the voices quoted in this chapter reflect general public concerns, they do not always translate into a patient's disquiet with, or lack of trust in, their own personal doctor. Nevertheless, the question has to be asked whether this is changing. Have the responses of the medical profession to public concerns about medical values and professionalism been too limited in scope? To what extent does the profession appreciate that perceptions of professionalism are not fixed in time, and that public expectations change? Has the profession been sufficiently *proactive* in recognising that public hopes and needs may have to be part of a new professionalism? Such hopes and needs are considered in the following chapters, while at the same time asking whether individual physicians can fulfil all public expectations.

Endnotes

1 Quoted in Huth EJ and Murray TJ (eds) (2000) *Medicine in Quotations: views of health and disease through the ages.* American College of Physicians, Philadelphia, p. 227.

2 For example, Creuss RL and Creuss SR (1997) Teaching medicine as a profession in the service of healing. *Academic Medicine.* **72**: 941–52. For a clear sense of growing change in the late 1990s, see Gray S (ed) (2003) *The 30th Anniversary Lectures Series, Faculty of Medicine.* Memorial University of Newfoundland, St John's (various invitational lectures).

3 Misch DA (2002) Evaluating physicians' professionalism and humanism: the case for humanism 'connoisseurs'. *Academic Medicine.* **77**: 489–95. This American comment is apt for elsewhere. For an illustrative discussion on teaching professionalism, Martin J, Lloyd M and Singh S (2002) Professional attitudes: can they be taught and assessed in medical education? *Clinical Medicine Journal of the Royal College of Physicians of London.* **2**: 217–23.

4 Earning trust is increasingly noted in the medical literature, e.g. Coulter A (2002) Patients' views of the good doctor. Doctors have to earn patients' trust. *British Medical Journal.* **325**: 668–9.

5 Published in *The Telegram* [St John's], 18 February 1999.

6 The relevant sociological literature is vast; some is contradictory, but the characteristics noted above are generally recognised. Much of the discussion on medical professionalism, especially by sociologists, is set in the context of physician power. For a thoughtful account of medical power, Howard Brody's (1992) *The Healer's Power*, Yale University Press, New Haven, notes that its various tentacles must be recognised in all areas of medical practice as a core issue in medical ethics. Brody describes three forms of doctors' power: (i) aesculapian power that rests on specialised knowledge and skills and the privileges, accorded by society, such that practitioners are allowed to investigate intimately the body in health, illness and death; (ii) charismatic power reflecting a practitioner's personality; and (iii) social power from status and roles in society. The latter, in particular, has been questioned by society in recent decades.

7 Harper HH (1930) *Merely the Patient.* Minton, Balch & Company, New York, pp. 36–8 for quote and quotes below.

8 Cf. Burnham JC (1982) American medicine's golden age: what happened to it? *Science.* **215**: 1474–9. For another account raising questions about the time parameters of the golden age, Brandt AM and Gardner M (2000) The golden age of medicine. In: Cooter R and Pickstone J (eds) *Medicine in the Twentieth Century.* Harwood Academic Publishing, Amsterdam, pp. 21–37.

A by-way of medical history, relevant not only to this period, is the creation of medical heroes within popular culture. A particularly interesting aspect of this is the role of comic books; see Hansen B (2004) Medical history for the masses: how American comic books celebrated heroes of medicine in the 1940s. *Bulletin of the History of Medicine.* **78**: 148–91. Of particular interest, too, Vipond M (1982) A Canadian hero of the 1920s: Dr Frederick G Banting. *Canadian Historical Review.* **63**: 461–86.

9   The early decades of the century witnessed what has been called the patient-as-a-person movement. See Shorter E (1996) Primary care. In: Porter R (ed) *The Cambridge Illustrated History of Medicine.* Cambridge University Press, Cambridge, pp. 118–53.

10 The comments here on Rachel Carson rely on Leopold E (1999) *A Darker Ribbon: breast cancer, women and their doctors in the twentieth century.* Beacon Press, Boston, pp. 111–50.

11 Ibid., p. 130 for quote. Nowadays one can hear of the use of language that skirts around malignancy, e.g. people who have a 'touch' of cancer.

12 Ibid., p. 132.

13 Caston A (1997) *Flying Out With the Wounded.* New York University Press, New York, pp. 12–14.

14 Evocative images from poets became fairly well known in the nineteenth century, in large part through William Ernest Henley. His experiences in the Edinburgh Infirmary were captured in a series of 'Hospital Sketches', the first of which appeared in 1875. For overview: Baron JH (1988) Professor Lord Lister, William Ernest Henley, and Oscar Wilde. *British Medical Journal.* **297**: 1651–3.

15 Particularly provoking views include surrealist paintings by Frida Kahlo and the cult movie, *Tales from the Grimli Hospital* (1988). The latter is about two patients confined together during a smallpox epidemic in turn-of-the-century Grimli, Manitoba, Canada; their unconventional behaviour and treatment highlights the disturbing world of hospitals. Community pride in hospitals can be documented in various ways, but one of special interest is postcards with scenes of hospitals and often with 'booster captions' on the address side.

16 For movies as a medical humanities resource and their use in this volume, see Chapter 1 endnote 42.

17 For discussion on Kildare, including television sequels, Turow J (1989) *Television, Storytelling and Medical Power.* Oxford University Press, New York, pp. 7–26; Kalisch PA and Kalisch BJ (1985) When Americans called for Dr Kildare: images of physicians and nurses in the Dr Kildare and Dr Gillespie movies, 1937–1947. *Medical Heritage.* Sept/Oct: 348–63; Dans PE (2000) *Doctors in the Movies. Boil the Water and Just Say Aah.* Medi-Ed Press, Bloomington, pp. 64–74. One of the testimonials to Dr Kildare as a role model for a career in medicine is found in Floyd P Garrett, MD, Interview and Frequently Asked Questions: www.bma-wellness.com/aboutus/Garrett_Interview.html (accessed July 2004).

    For movie depictions of psychiatrists, Chapter 10. For ophthalmologists cf. *Blink* (1994) and for obstetricians, *The Hand that Rocks the Cradle* (1992).

18 Many a physician, however, questions the movie *Patch Adams*; see Dans, *Doctors in the Movies. Boil the Water and Just Say Aah*, pp. 21–8. Patch Adams' provocative writings include (1998) *House Calls: how we can all heal the sick one visit at a time*, Robert Reed, San Francisco (also challenges hospital visitors to consider how they may help heal the person they visit), and (1998) *Gesundheit*, Healing Arts Press, Rochester, Vermont. In a contrasting way, a 2003 Canadian movie, *The Barbarian Invasions*, challenges patient care in the Canadian healthcare system, and adds to concerns in the US and UK.

19 For censorship: Shortland M (1989) *Medicine and Film: a checklist, survey and research resource.* Wellcome Unit for the History of Medicine, Oxford, pp. 8–9; Lederer SE (1998) Repellent subjects: Hollywood censorship and surgical images in the 1930s. *Literature and Medicine.* **17**: 91–113. Censorship took many forms. A noteworthy example is the hospital murder mystery, *Green for Danger* (1946), which was temporarily banned in Britain on the grounds that a wounded soldier seeing the film might have their recovery slowed for fear of being murdered in hospital. (Shortland [this note] p. 32.)

20 Images over time, especially caricatures and cartoons, not only lampoon physicians, but also offer much social commentary as well as documenting trends in medicine. Cf. Porter R (2001) *Bodies Politic. Disease, Death and Doctors in Britain.* Cornell University Press,

Ithaca, which makes clear that charges of questionable physician morals, such as happened in the second half of the twentieth century, were not new. Also, Helfand WH (1990) A less than loving look at doctors. *1991 Medical and Health Annual*. Encyclopedia Britannica, Chicago, pp. 22–39. However, the intensity of the public and media questioning of physicians has changed.

21   For philosophical discussion on playing God as a pejorative label, Erde EL (1989) Studies in the explanation of issues in biomedial ethics. (II) 'On play[ing] God', etc. *Journal of Medicine and Philosophy*. **14**: 593–615. Although the public knows little about the story of Hippocrates, his oath has contributed much to him becoming viewed as the ideal physician.

A short story by physician Michael LaCombe, 'Playing God', merits mention as an example of real dilemmas facing physicians. The story is about a physician called out by a patient who tells him, 'My husband has passed away, Doctor. Can you come over?' The caller is a long-time patient abused by her husband over many years, but who repeatedly goes back to him. The physician finds that the wife, now with a broken arm, has shot the husband though she claims he shot himself. The physician rearranges the scene to make it look like a suicide. Legal responsibilities are clear, but there remains much to debate about ethical/legal boundaries, the real dilemmas that occur in everyday practice, and whether playing God can ever be justified. LaCombe MA (1992) Playing God. *Annals of Internal Medicine*. **116**: 161–2. For comments by a physician, Cassel CK 'Reflections on Playing God'. ibid., pp. 163–4; 'Playing God – Revisited' (Letters to Editor), ibid., p. 1035.

22   Winchester S (1967) *The Practice*. Putnam's Sons, New York.

23   Ibid., p. 135.

24   Kaye D (1993) *Laugh, I Thought I'd Die. My Life with ALS*. Penguin Books Canada, Toronto, p. 46.

25   For an example of a reawakening, see Dr Michael Reynolds in *Sunchaser* (1996); early on in the kidnapping of Reynolds by a 16-year-old patient in search of an aboriginal healer, the youth shouted at him: 'I got you down as God.'

26   Although a substantial literature exists on near-death experiences, agreement exists that more studies are needed. For general review, Greyson B (1991) Encounters with death. *1992 Medical and Health Annual*. Encyclopedia Britannica, Chicago, pp. 46–55.

27   Publication figures given in Wear D (2002) The house of God: another look. *Academic Medicine*. **77**: 496–501. The book had a lukewarm reception from the medical profession with various attempts to discredit it. Wear critically discusses existing appraisals and Shem's view that the novel is controversial because it tells the 'truth'.

28   Shem S (1995) *The House of God*. Dell Publishing, New York, introduction unpaginated.

29   Anon. (2003) Physician writers: Samuel Shem. *Lancet*. **361**: 536. See also Shem S (2002) Fiction as resistance. *Annals of Internal Medicine*. **137**: 934–7.

30   Shem S (1997) *Mount Misery*. Fawcett Columbine, New York. Shem's real name, Stephen Bergman, is revealed.

31   For one view on the role of humanity and idealism, Marion R (1992) *Learning to Play God: the coming of age of a young doctor*. Addison-Wesley, Reading, Massachusetts, p. xvi and dust jacket for quote.

32   From Maurya Simon, The AIDS Ward, USC Medical Center. In: Mukand J (ed) (1994) *Articulations: the body and illness in poetry*. University of Iowa Press, Iowa City, p. 43.

33   From George Garrett, In the Hospital, ibid., p. 31.

34   Thompson JD and Goldin G (1975) *The Hospital: a social and architectural history*. Yale University Press, New Haven, p. 189.

35   Information from postcards mailed in the 1930s (author's collection). Judging from the relatively large number of such cards depicting the Medical Center, still available to collectors, it was considered one of the more striking features of New York.

36   Postcard (author's collection), published by *Health Matters*, reporting on 'today's NHS [National Health Service] and public health issues'. Website: www.healthmatters. org.uk (accessed May 2003).

37   For some context to issues, see Bulger RE and Reiser SJ (eds) (1990) *Integrity in Health Care Institutions: humane environments for teaching, inquiry, and healing*. University of Iowa, Iowa City. For example, Rozovsky L (1994) *The Canadian Patient's Book of Rights: a consumer's guide to Canadian health law*. Doubleday Canada, Toronto.

38 The patient examines the doctor. In: Broyard A (1992) *Intoxicated By My Illness and Other Writings on Life and Death.* Clarkson Potter, New York, p. 35.
39 Lawrence M (1964) *The Stone Angel.* University of Chicago Press, Chicago, quotes from pp. 88–93. The novel describes the life of Hagar Shipley, who tells of her present condition as she attempts to avoid her son and daughter-in-law who want to put her in a nursing home. Another interesting waiting-room scene appears in Winckler M (2000) *The Case of Dr Sachs.* Seven Stories, New York, p. 309.

> Beside me, the teenager and her mother keep needling one another. Or rather, the mother is needling the girl with her 'You'll see, I'm going to tell him. We can't just leave you like this. It can't go on. I'm doing this for your own sake, you know! After all, I *am* your mother.' And the girl answers, 'Stop it! Stop it, you're driving me crazy!' and keeps sighing endlessly. The door opens. The man with the cap comes out: 'Good, well, can't take up your time! People are waiting for you! So, okay, good-bye then, Doctor, see you in a month!'

40 Broyard, *Intoxicated by my Illness*, p. 35. Comments about offices have been long-standing. In 1842, physician Daniel Drake, for example, in exhorting medical students to develop good practice, expressed concerns that were to be respeated time and time again: 'Who can read and think, with method or sound logic, while everything around him is dirty and disordered? His little stock of furniture displaced, as if a riot had just passed away; his books scattered on chairs, tables, and the greasy medicine shelves; in his book cases, volumes of different sets mixed together, some lying flat, and some, like the ideas of their reader, upside down.' Quoted in Crellin JK and Pearson EF (1977) Currents/Crosscurrents [on physicians' offices]. *Aspects. Quarterly Journal of Southern Illinois University Medical School.* **1** (2): 14–16.
41 For an invaluable introduction to pictures of medical practice, including doctors' offices and waiting-rooms, Stoekle JD and White GA (1985) *Plain Pictures of Plain Doctoring: vernacular expression in new deal medicine.* MIT Press, Cambridge. In 'reading' a photograph various questions need to be asked. Is the photograph merely a frozen instant of time? Is it candid and uncontrived, or is it a posed 'set-up?' Whose vision are we seeing? That is, from whose point of view is the photograph taken? Was the photograph intended for any particular purpose? Is there an intended message? Is it propaganda? Is there anything in the photograph that may not be part of the intended message? What is not shown? Are photographs the 'truth'? For these and other issues, and many photographs, see Fox DM and Lawrence C (1988) *Photographing Medicine: images and power in Britain and America since 1840.* Greenwood Press, New York.
42 Personal communication, Nancie Rideout.
43 London O (1987) *Kill as Few Patients as Possible, and Fifty-Six Other Essays on How to Be the World's Best Doctor.* Ten Speed Press, Berkeley, p. 5 (under 'Rule 2: Have a Lovely Office').
44 Schneider GW and Dehaven MJ (2003) Revising the Navaho way: lessons for contemporary healing. *Perspectives in Biology and Medicine.* **46**: 413–27 (423).
45 For various views: Russell PC (2002) The white coat ceremony: turning trust into entitlement. *Teaching and Learning in Medicine.* **14**: 56–9; Huber SJ (2003) The white coat ceremony: a contemporary medical ritual. *Journal of Medical Ethics.* **29**: 364–6; Glick SM (2003) White coat ceremonies: another commentary. *Journal of Medical Ethics.* **29**: 367–8; Panja A (2004) The death of the white coat. *British Medical Journal.* **328**: 57.
    Feelings exist that a sense of 'belonging' to the profession is less easy for many students today than in the past. Far fewer have parents who are physicians; and many students, especially in North America, attend relatively new medical schools with little or no tradition. Moreover, most students are not exposed to sufficient history of medicine to have a good understanding of their medical roots, even of the nature of the Hippocratic oath that they are likely to take on graduation. It is noteworthy that in North America, medical schools in which students take the Hippocratic oath grew to 100 percent in the 1990s. (Crawshaw R (2003) Swearing medical oaths, 1999. *The Pharos.* Winter: 33–5.)
46 Brandt LJ (2003) On the value of an old dress code in the new millennium. *Archives of Internal Medicine.* **163**: 1277–81.

47 The 1990s saga in Britain of multiple murders by general practitioner Harold Shipman (designated 'Dr Death' by the media), which aroused tremendous public concern, was also a reminder that many physicians have been serial or single victim murderers. One commentator has said 'Arguably medicine has thrown up more serial killers than all the other professions put together.' Kinnell HG (2000) Serial homicide by doctors: Shipman in perspective. *British Medical Journal.* **321**: 1594–7. Also, Iverson KV (2002) *Demon Doctors: physicians as serial killers.* Galen Press, Tucson.

48 The issue of unnecessary hysterectomies can be seen in the context of claims of other unnecessary surgeries, which, in recent years, have come from insurance companies as well as patients. For early general discussion, 'Unnecessary Surgery' in Sharpe VA and Faden AI (1988) *Medical Harm: historical, conceptual, and ethical dimensions of iatrogenic illness.* Cambridge University Press, Cambridge, pp. 194–209.

It should be noted that media coverage is not always easy to interpret as it can embrace both acceptance of the power of physician expertise and the risks physicians face in the hands of patients. (See Bradby H, Gabe J and Bury M (1995) 'Sexy docs' and 'busty blondes': press coverage of professional misconduct cases brought before the General Medical Council. *Sociology of Health & Illness.* **17**: 458–76.) Bizarre cases colour the entire scene as when an obstetrician – ultimately diagnosed with mental disabilities – carved his initials on the abdomen of a patient on whom he had performed a caesarean section. For one of many reports on this, with a somewhat embroidered heading: Andrusko D 'Probation for New York Abortionist who Carved Initials into Maternity Patient's Abdomen': www.nrlc.org/news/2000/NRL05/zarkin.html (accessed July 2004).

49 I am grateful to Pam Hall for this observation.

50 The account of the story around Dr John Schneeberger, working in a rural Saskatchewan hospital: www.cbc.ca/stories/1999/11/26/Saskdr9911267 (accessed December 2003).

51 This is an aspect of doctors getting 'knocked off the pedestal', for which see Dans PE (2000) *Doctors in the Movies. Boil the Water and Just say Aah.* Medi-Ed Press, Bloomington, pp. xviii–xxii.

52 Ibid., p. 222.

53 Shem (1995) *The House of God,* pp. 11–12.

54 Dans *Doctors in the Movies,* pp. 121–47. Chapter on 'Where Are All the Woman Doctors'.

55 In *The Prince of Tides,* sex takes place with a patient's relative, though the relative can also be viewed as the patient as can the psychiatrist, but the misuse of physician power remains an issue. For discussion on *Coma, The Prince of Tides* and other films with women physicians, Dans' *Doctors in the Movies,* pp. 121–47. Dans concludes that women doctors 'have been, for the most part, weak or inordinately submissive' (p. 147).

56 Conley FK (1998) *Walking Out on the Boys.* Farrar, Straus and Giroux, New York. A substantial autobiographical literature by women exists, much of it offering corrections to stereotypes. For some introduction, Sirridge MS and Pfannenstiel BR (1996) Daughters of Aesculapius: a selected bibliography of autobiographies of women medical school graduates, 1849–1920. *Literature and Medicine.* **15**: 200–16. See also Women Physicians' Autobiographies: www.research.med.umkc.edu/teams/cml/womendrs.html (accessed July 2004).

57 Masters EL (1976) *Spoon River Anthology.* Collier, New York, p. 46 (originally published 1915). Mrs Meyers, from the graveyard (p. 47) makes clear her husband had broken 'the law human and divine'.

58 Williams WC (1996) Old Doc Rivers. In: *The Collected Stories of William Carlos Williams.* A New Directions Book, New York, pp. 77–105 (p. 104 for quote). See also Williams J and Schneiderman H (1988) The ethics of impaired physicians: Wolfe's Dr McGuire and William's Dr Rivers. *Literature and Medicine.* **7**: 123–31. Oral histories from elder physicians suggest that there have been many 'models' for fictional alcoholic practitioners.

59 Saunders GL (1994) *Doctor Olds of Twillingate: portrait of an American surgeon in Newfoundland.* St John's, Breakwater, p. 169, italics added. From the chapter 'Alcohol'.

60 This story comes from the early twentieth century. I am grateful to Dr Ian Rusted for the information.

61 Davies R (1970) *Fifth Business.* Macmillan, Toronto.

62 Shem (1995) *The House of God*, p. 14. Gomer is defined as 'Get Out of My Emergency Room, "a human being who has lost – often through age – what goes into being a human being".'

63 For the question, How did he hide this from colleagues? Olch PD (1975) William S Halsted and local anaesthesia. *Anaesthesiology.* **42**: 479–86.

64 From James Tate, On the subject of doctors. In: Mukand J (ed) (1994) *Articulations: the body and illness in poetry*. University of Iowa Press, Iowa City, p. 134.

65 For physician perspectives on stresses: Gorlin R, Strain J and Rhodes R (1996) Physicians' reactions to patients: what has happened during the past 10 years. *The Mount Sinai Journal of Medicine.* **63**: 420–4.

66 Cf. Gifford GE (1973) Fildes and the 'The Doctor'. *Journal of the American Medical Association.* **224**: 61–3. As an icon image: Connor JTH, unpublished lecture on the influence of the picture. For other pictures, Emery AEH and Emery MLH (2003) *Medicine and Art*. Royal Society of Medicine Press, London. A review of this book by A Borsay (2003) points up different interpretations, *Medical Humanities Edition of the Journal Medical Ethics.* **29**: 108.

67 See Barilan YM (2004) Medicine through the artist's eyes before, during, and after the holocaust. *Perspectives in Biology and Medicine.* **47**: 110–34.

68 Many items are, in fact, frank nostalgia rather than offering serious historical perspective. If a comprehensive bibliography of rural doctors existed, it would be extensive (many from small local presses), for there seems to be an insatiable appetite among the public. A noteworthy museum for its theme, The Country Doctor Museum in Bailey, North Carolina, USA, is dedicated to the goal of 'honouring' the old country doctor, as do exhibits in many small museums.
    Country docs appear in a wide range of novels, sometimes as the saviour of a community. A press release for William T Close's 2002 *Subversion of Trust* (Meadowlark Springs Productions, Big Piney) asks 'Are today's doctors cogs in the medical industry or physicians we can trust?' www.williamtclosemd.com/subversion.html (accessed July 2004). The character Alex McKinnon, an elder rural doc, is the hero. A more significant influence has been the television series, *Dr Quinn, Medicine Woman*, see www.drquinnmd.com (accessed July 2004).

69 The historical record points up the hardships of practice in many ways; for instance, the account book of James A Russell, a North Carolina doctor, noted on 8 September 1846 that he charged a family $10, but that the cost would be $4 provided the physician was not sent for in the night soon after having passed his house. (Crellin JK, The Everyday Setting and Practice of a Physician, unpublished manuscript.) One particular frustration for physicians was that a difficult housecall might turn out to be for a very minor one, albeit one worrying the patient. For a revealing physician's journal – distinct from recollections – that points up the real hardships of rural practice, especially in cold winters: Ecke RS (2000) *Snowshoe & Lancet. Memoirs of a frontier Newfoundland doctor 1947–1948*. Rendall, Portsmouth, New Hampshire.

70 Dans (2000) *Doctors in the Movies*, p. 37. Dafoe acquired widespread media publicity that included postcards showing him with the quins.

71 Dowling GF (1998) What makes a good doctor? Practicing medicine the old fashioned way. *Life.* **21** (17): 48–52.

72 Loxterkamp D (1997) *A Measure of My Days: the journal of a country doctor*. University Press of New England, Hanover.

73 Ibid., p. 3.

74 Pocius GL (1991) *A Place to Belong: community order and everyday space in Calvert, Newfoundland*. University of Georgia Press, Athens/McGill-Queen's University Press, Montreal.

75 Berger and Mohr (1967) *The Story of a Country Doctor*. The Penguin Press, London.

76 The influence of the movie *Whose Life is it Anyway* is based on an earlier play, and the phrase itself can be best seen through a Google search (225 000 hits July 2004).

77 A key feature of the film is that Harrison's physicians labelled his wish to die as 'depression'; other health professionals, less certain of the diagnostic label, categorised him as a difficult patient. Some physicians continue to see only compliant patients as 'model' patients.

78 Atwood M (1982) *Bodily Harm*. Simon & Schuster, New York. Summary from pp. 32–5.

79 Handler E (1996) *Time on Fire: my comedy of terror*. Little Brown, Boston. Summary below from pp. 272–8.

80 Brody H (2003) *Stories of Sickness*. Oxford University Press, Toronto, pp. 262–5.

81 For annotated and general bibliographies of academic analyses up to 1995, see American Board of Internal Medicine, *Project Professionalism*; most recent printing available online at www.abim.org, pp. 31–41 (accessed July 2004).

82 Lown B (1996) *The Lost Art of Healing*. Houghton Mifflin, Boston, p. xi.

83 Lundberg G (2000) *Severed Trust: why American medicine hasn't been fixed*. Basic Books, New York, p. 155.

84 Much of the recent writings on professionalism stresses the need to preserve the values of compassion, trust, honesty and integrity. It seems appropriate in a book on voices to notice a few examples of historical writings that have been significant amid the constant exhortations for physicians to sustain long-standing professional values. All serve as a reminder that relationships with patients have always been an issue for physicians and have been approached in various ways. Thomas Percival (1803), in his far-reaching *Medical Ethics* (Johnson and Bickerstaff, Manchester, pp. 10–11), wrote: 'The feelings and emotions of the patients under critical circumstances, require to be known and to be attended to, no less than the symptoms of their diseases ... Even the *prejudices* of the sick are not to be condemned, or opposed with harshness. For though silenced by authority, they will operate secretly and forcibly on the mind, creating fear, anxiety, and watchfulness.'

In contrast, Oliver Wendell Holmes (1883) expressed the epitomy of paternalism in 'The Young Practitioner' (*Medical Essays 1842–1882*. Houghton Mifflin, Boston, pp. 388–9): 'Your patient has no more right to all the truth you know than he has to all the medicine in your saddle-bags, if you carry that kind of cartridge-box for the ammunition that slays disease. He should get only just so much as is good for him ... Some shrewd old doctors have a few phrases always on hand for patients that will insist on knowing the pathology of their complaints without the slightest capacity of understanding the scientific explanation. I have known the term "spinal irritation" serve well on such occasions, but I think nothing on the whole has covered so much ground, and meant so little, and given such profound satisfaction to all parties, as the magnificent phrase "congestion of the portal system".'

Daniel Webster Cathell (1882) *The Physician Himself and What He Should Add to His Scientific Acquirements*. Cushings and Bailey, Baltimore (p. 102): 'When a sick person puts himself under your care he gives you a responsible duty to perform. If he then neglects or refuses to take your remedies he ties your hands and keeps you from doing it. If, however, he will not or cannot do exactly as you wish, and if no special danger exists, it is sometimes better, after drawing attention to the position in which you are placed (as a protection to yourself), to humor his whims or weaknesses, and modify or alter your therapeutics to such things as he can and will do. This you can do good-naturedly without fully yielding to him or compromising your authority or your dignity. The wishes, prejudices and errors of peculiar patients must be studied and to a certain extent respected.'

William Peabody (1930) *Doctor and Patient*. Macmillan, New York (pp. 32–3): 'Everybody, sick or well, is affected in one way or another, consciously or subconsciously, by the material and spiritual forces that bear on his life, and especially to the sick such forces may act as powerful stimulants or depressants. When the general practitioner goes into the home of a patient, he may know the whole background of the family life from past experience; but even when he comes as a stranger he has every opportunity to find out what manner of man his patient is, and what kind of circumstances makes his life ... When a patient enters a hospital, the first thing that commonly happens to him is that he loses his personal identity. He is generally referred to, not as Henry Jones, but as "that case of mitral stenosis in the second bed on the left".'

85 LaCombe MA (1993) On professionalism. *American Journal of Medicine*. **94**: 329. See also his story (1996) Problems of professionalization: physician impairment. *American Journal of Medicine*. **101**: 654–6, for an account of stresses leading to a loss of professionalism.

86 Cf. Irvine D (2001) Doctors in the UK: their new professionalism and its regulatory framework. *Lancet*. **358**: 1807–10. It is appropriate to note that the British medical

profession, stunned by such events as the deaths of many children following surgery at the Bristol Royal Infirmary between 1984 and 1995, and the multiple murders by general practitioner Harold Shipman (already noted), has faced vigorous demands for greater public accountability. Traditionally, British medicine has not dwelt on Codes of Ethics to the same extent as has the profession in North America. However, since the late 1990s, the booklet *Good Medical Practice* is circulated to newly registered practitioners in the UK. It includes the following statement of 'duties and responsibilities of doctors':

> Patients must be able to trust doctors with their lives and well-being. To justify that trust, we as a profession have a duty to maintain a good standard of practice and care and to show respect for human life. In particular as a doctor you must: make the care of your patient your first concern; treat every patient politely and considerately; respect patients' dignity and privacy; listen to patients and respect their views; give patients information in a way they can understand; respect the rights of patients to be fully involved in decisions about their care; keep your professional knowledge and skills up to date; recognise the limits of your professional competence; be honest and trustworthy; respect and protect confidential information; make sure that your personal beliefs do not prejudice your patients' care; act quickly to protect patients from risk if you have good reason to believe that you or a colleague may not be fit to practise; avoid abusing your position as a doctor; and work with colleagues in the ways that best serve patients' interests. (*Good Medical Practice* (3e) (2001) General Medical Council, London, p. 2.)

87   Listed in (2002) Medical professionalism in the new millennium: a physician charter. *Annals of Internal Medicine.* **136**: 243–6.
88   American Board of Internal Medicine, *Project Professionalism.* Available: www.abim. org/pubs/p2/ (accessed July 2004).
89   Ibid., p. 1.
90   For one US response: Klein EJ, Jackson JC, Kratz L *et al.* (2003) Teaching professionalism to residents. *Academic Medicine.* **78**: 26–34.
91   Wear D and Nixon LL (2002) Literary inquiry and professional development in medicine. Against abstractions. *Perspectives in Biology and Medicine.* **45**: 104–24.
92   Campo R (1997) *The Poetry of Healing: a doctor's education, empathy, identity and desire.* Norton, New York, p. 140.
93   Shem S (1997) *Mount Misery.* Fawcett Columbine, New York, p. 64.

CHAPTER 3

Communication and the art of medicine

Proper communication is one of the most difficult undertakings on earth. The older I get, the more I am forced to recognize that many breakdowns and tragedies have their origin in faulty communications ... In the medical world, you need go no further than the administration of hospital affairs to see how many errors, some of them serious, proceed from faulty communications. Consider the wrong medications in the intravenous bottle or the wrong pills or the wrong quantities, or the hospital attendant who mistakenly interprets instructions. Not infrequently, that attendant can point to ambiguous communications. The orders just weren't clear enough. (Norman Cousins)[1]

Growing interest in 'medical communication', particularly since the 1970s, has been driven by countless stories of poor physician communication, by new legal and ethical underpinnings of informed consent, and by growing emphasis on patient-centred care. Vigorous voices like Norman Cousins, a spokesperson for countless patients, along with extensive social science research, have focused particular attention on communication as the heart of effective physician–patient relationships.[2] Cousins adds to the above quote that, in his contacts with patients, he had been made aware of the frequency with which they seem frightened, confused or immobilised as the result of encounters with healthcare practitioners. He acknowledges that one problem may be their own failures in understanding, but he was nevertheless struck by the frequent impairment of patient and physician relationships because of careless communication.

It can come as no surprise that the public should specify, indeed challenge, the medical profession to ensure that a central role for a physician is as a communicator. Of many relevant issues, this chapter notices just two key ones that emerge as strong messages from the voices of humanities; they are (1) the barriers of medical terminology (a 'foreign' language) and (2) the failures of physicians to listen to patients. The voices, too, also offer, sometimes indirectly, suggestions about how physicians might respond.

Growing communication difficulties

Robertson Davies wrote thoughtfully about talking with patients in his novel *The Cunning Man* (1994). In the words of his main character, Dr Jonathan Hullah, he views doctors as 'men of substantial education, though not always men of wide culture'. He adds: 'they develop a manner, and a vocabulary suitable to their professional status, which is sufficient in civilian life, and which is often reassuring to the uneducated patient.'[3] However, in noting that sick and wounded men in World War II, who are in a strange land, 'need another kind of talk', Davies seems to be asking physicians to consider the needs of *individual* patients who find themselves in the 'strange land' of medical care. What is needed is 'friendly, not patronizing or simple talk, but that which inspires trust in men'.

Communication barriers are not new. A brief look at general trends, beginning with the nineteenth century, indicates something of the various ways communication difficulties have arisen, been ignored, or otherwise approached by physicians. Indeed, maybe communication problems should be approached as an endemic disease of medicine.

During the 1800s, physicians often sidestepped communication difficulties. Physician–writer Oliver Wendell Holmes told students in 1871 that 'some shrewd old doctors have a few phrases always on hand for patients that will insist on knowing the pathology of their complaints without the slightest capacity of understanding the scientific explanation.'[4] This strategy was presumably implemented even when the social standing of patients made it clear that they were 'employers' of a doctor. Well known to those who enjoy classic nineteenth-century novels is Anthony Trollope's *Dr Thorne* (1858). Trollope illuminates factors of class, medical hierarchies and marital status relevant to physician–patient relationships at the time. He makes clear the employer role of patients, but nevertheless that the medical authority of the doctor had to be acknowledged. This is evident in the relationship Dr Thorne developed with Sir Roger Scatcherd, as indicated in the following banter:

'It's natural she [your wife] should be anxious about your health, you know.'

'I don't know that,' said the contractor [Scatcherd]. 'She'll be very well off. All that whining won't keep a man alive, at any rate.'

There was a pause, during which the doctor continued his medical examination. To this the patient submitted with a bad grace, but still he did submit.

'We must turn over a new leaf Sir Roger; indeed we must.'

'Bother,' said Sir Roger.

'Well Scatcherd; I must do my duty to you, whether you like it or not.'

'That is to say, I am to pay you for trying to frighten me.'[5]

There is no doubt that, at the time (mid-nineteenth century onward), communicating the nature of medical problems in terms of the new clinico-pathological approach to understanding disease – that is, correlating signs and symptoms of a disease with post-mortem, chemical and clinical observations – was increasingly a challenge. For one thing, by finally displacing long-standing humoral notions, diseases came to be viewed more often in terms of anatomical rather than functional changes;[6] this shift eclipsed much of the sense of understanding between patients and doctors, for humoral-related explanations had long been part of general, not just physicians', culture. William Osler summarised a changing situation in 1889: 'from the standpoint of medicine as an art for the prevention and the cure of the disease, the man who translates the hieroglyphics of science into the plain language of healing is certainly the more useful.'[7]

Translation difficulties were compounded by the nineteenth-century avalanche of diagnostic tools that 'observed' and measured the pathology: stethoscopes, chemical testing of urine, self-registering thermometers, sphygmomanometers for measuring blood pressure, X-rays, etc. Apart from introducing a new vocabulary, such technology refashioned how case histories were taken, and thereby physician–patient communication. Consultations became more a series of questions and answers to add to information obtained through a physical examination. Listening to a patient's account of their conditions assumed less importance for the physician. Comments to students (published 1878), by a highly respected clinician Peter Latham, illuminate changing medical approaches even without specific mention of instruments.

> Now, in taking the case, I desire always to proceed after a certain method; and, when I am able to pursue that method, all the circumstances which I seek to know unfold themselves naturally and easily, and then it is a simple, agreeable, and interesting employment.
>
> But often, very often, I am driven from all pretence of method in taking the case. The poor patient is embarrassed by the novelty of his situation, or he is deaf, or his disease incapacitates him; and he hardly understands your questions, and gives you strange answers. Thus things drop out confusedly one after another, and you must be content to accept them as they come, and join them together as you can. But, upon these terms, taking a case becomes a very irksome, disagreeable business.[8]

Latham went on to say that he asks no questions 'until I have learned everything worthy of remark which my own eyes can inform me of'. This was followed by 'further inquiry in which the patient takes a part', namely, systematic questioning about general sensations and particular organs – eyes, chest, heart, etc.

Amidst the nineteenth-century trends, many patients began to feel like 'black boxes' – a sentiment that persists. In 1892, a patient complained of the artificial bearing of a physician in a sick room and the big scientific words that rolled off the tongue.[9] Not surprisingly, the following years up to the 1960s were hardly noted for *effective* dialogue between physicians and patients. In general, patients asked few questions about the details of their care; a physician's authority was rarely challenged, at least openly, unless it contradicted that of another physician. Cartoonists, however, found riches in miscommunication, much of it in line with the long history of spotlighting and pricking the pomposity of doctors. Medical malapropisms – a patient's mispronounciation of a medical term, or misinterpreting it as a common word – often appeared on comic postcards.[10] One, mailed in 1909, shows a country wife talking to her ailing husband: 'Yerself ought to be a proud man to-night. The doctors say ye have bad information [inflammation] on the brain with severe indigestion [congestion] of the lungs and a touch of new-mown hay [pneumonia] which may at any minuit turn to a guitar [catarrh] of yer pedestrian [respiration] organs, so he is coming to telescope [stethoscope] ye to-morrow.'

And another card, mailed 1932, depicted a working-class woman who confused an 'opening medicine' (a laxative) with an 'opium' medicine, many of which were still sold over the counter at the time.

Aside from malapropisms, total misunderstandings of medical directions were depicted. For instance:

The medicine hadn't worked

Doctor: 'Did ye take the box of pills I sent you?'

Patient: 'Ooh! Doctor dear, I did, but I misdoubt the lid hasn't come off yet.'

(Postcard mailed 1908)

Doctor: 'Well, did you follow my advice and eat plenty of animal food?'

Patient: 'Yes Sir. I got on alright with the oats, but the chopped hay took a bit of getting down.'

(Postcard mailed 1912).

That such jokes, as far-fetched as they may seem, were not necessarily total figments of a cartoonist's imagination comes from a 1980s collection of malapropisms that included 'athletic' or 'electrical' fits (epileptic fits), 'electric lights' (electrolytes), 'telescoped' (fluoroscoped), 'monogram' (myelogram), 'terrible clombosis' (cerebral thrombosis), and 'vultures' (convulsions).[11] Moreover, many testimonies exist that patients, when using suppositories for the first time, fail to remove the foil wrapping. It is appropriate to notice that communication nowadays is hardly helped by the increasing use of abbreviations and acronyms. Although some such as DNR and D&C have become familiar through popular culture, the littering of medical discourse with, for example, CHF (congested heart failure), PFT (pulmonary function test) or even PSA (prostate-specific antigen) makes medical language even more inaccessible to patients.[12]

Physicians have to recognise the difficulties of medical terminology. Many try to avoid it, and sometimes end up talking down to a patient; indeed, non-medical language may even confuse a patient as suggested by another postcard cartoon published around 1925 – a time when popular medical texts constantly compared the body to an engine. The card shows a doctor with stethoscope listening to the chest of a bemused patient. The doctor tells him: 'Your resistance couplers are a bit wobbly. Your choke coil seems alright. But I think perhaps your grid leak would do with a clear out.'

Public concerns over poor communication became increasingly evident post 1950s. New sensitivities emerged to what was viewed as physician paternalism and arrogance. Movie repartee was underscoring this in the 1950s. In *Doctor in the House* (1954) – the first of a series of British medical comedies in the 1950s and '60s that provided audiences with a sense that patients could exercise their power – consultant physician Sir Lancelot Spratt, while bedside teaching, cavalierly told a hospital patient: 'Don't worry my good man, you won't understand our medical talk.' And, a hypochondriacal patient, in *Sunday Bloody Sunday* (1972), whose alarm at the suggestion of having some tests for abdominal pain prompts the following exchange.

> [Doctor]: 'Listen old friend, it's not cancer.'
> 'How do you know?'
> 'Because I'm telling you.'

Perhaps, however, invoking physician paternalism in the latter case was sound strategy for the 'old friend'.

A staccato exchange in *The Practice* (1967) captures how physicians may minimise dialogue and ignore 'difficult' questions, at least questions that would take up much physician time to respond adequately:[13]

> [Patient]: 'You don't think I ought to have an X-ray?'
>
> [Doctor]: 'An X-ray?'
>
> 'My mother's uncle died of cancer of the stomach.'
>
> 'I don't think you need worry about that, providing you've given me a full picture. No sign of blood in your stools?' He shook his head; Trevor [the physician] had a feeling he probably examined his stools with some care. 'Any vomiting? And the pains you get are three or four hours after you have eaten?'
>
> 'About that.'
>
> 'Then there's not the slightest reason to suspect a malignancy. I think you'll find these pills will do the trick. But we'll make an appointment for you to see Dr Knight [the patient's regular physician] again in a few days, as well.'
>
> He wrote out the prescription. While he was doing this, Lester [the patient] said, 'Doctor ... '
>
> 'Yes.'
>
> 'There's another thing.'
>
> 'What's that?'
>
> 'The way things are ... feeling so run down ... I don't always feel up to certain things.' He braced back his narrow shoulders. 'My marital duties.'
>
> 'Try not to worry about that. It's probably worry, more than anything else, that prevents you.'
>
> 'I have the feeling that my wife – well, wants more than I can give her.'
>
> 'Has she complained to you?'
>
> 'Oh, no!' He looked very shocked. 'She wouldn't do anything like that.'
>
> 'How often do you have intercourse?'
>
> 'Once a week. Sometimes only once a fortnight.'
>
> 'And how long have you been married?'

'Thirteen years.'

'Any children?'

'No.'

'Did you hope to have any?'

'We never felt the need.'

'Well, I shouldn't worry about your sexual relations with your wife. They're perfectly normal.'

Lester said something in a low voice, which Trevor did not catch. He said, 'I'm sorry – what was that?'

'She's very pretty.'

Trevor was slightly nonplussed. He said, 'Yes. Well, I think you'll find that these pills will put you on the right track. And can you get in to see Dr Knight on Friday?'

The exposure of questionable communication – sometimes attributed to practice situations circumscribed by the exigencies of healthcare insurance systems – has been very much part of a reconsideration of physician–patient relationships. New models of relationships, identified by such terms as 'collegial', 'contractual', and 'friendly', have been one consideration behind the push, in the 1990s, for formal medical education on communication. However, the question has to be asked whether the new trends adequately consider the long-standing gulf between lay and professional understanding of diseases and treatments. Although there can be no clear answer to this for some time, a sense exists that, in some medical schools at least, the new education focuses too exclusively on how best to elicit information in a limited consultation time, despite a recognition that effective communication is heavily dependent on the ability to explain technical language and, equally, to listen.

Listening to patients

> The doctor who sits at the bedside of a rat
> Obtains real answers – a paw twitch,
> An ear tremor, a gain or loss of weight,
> No problem as to which
> Is Temper and which is true
> What a rat feels, he will do
>
> Concomitantly then, the doctor who sits
> At the bedside of a rat
> Asks real questions, as befits
> the place, like where do that potassium go, not what
> Do you think of Willie Mays or the weather?
> So rat and doctor may converse together.
>
> (Josephine Miles, 1974)[14]

Going out of the surgery, clutching her bit of paper, a prescription for something at least, Daphne felt that Martin, the 'new doctor' as he was called in the village, had done her good. He had listened, he had been sympathetic and she felt decidedly better. Much better than she would have felt if she'd gone to Dr G – he never even bothered to take your blood pressure. (B Pym, 1980)[15]

In different ways, these two quotes are reminders that patients like Rachel Carson (*see* Chapter 2) have a real need to feel they are being listened to. Some see this as the essence of not being treated as a laboratory specimen. Increasingly since the 1970s, patients' concerns appear in their stories of experiences told to friends and neighbours and published accounts, often called autopathographies.[16] Notable earlier examples exist. In 1940, Duff Giffond describes what was perhaps familiar to many readers, namely, a physician not listening as he interrupts and short-circuits a patient's reply:

'What kind of a pain is it?' he [Dr Kelly] asked, with the interest of the doctor who isn't listening for a fee.

'Well, Doctor,' I replied, 'it feels like two quarts of stuff packed into a one-quart container.'

'Very good,' he snapped.'Exactly,' with a brisk turn to my friend, 'the kind of thing Senator Wanderding had. Ran around like crazy for three months until I took him to Dr Palmer. Fixed him up in no time there. And you know what it was?' he asked us, as we listened popeyed, hanging on his words. 'One little ingredient missing in his blood! Matter of finding it,' he concluded with a brisk wave of his hand, 'that's all.'

I was terribly excited. This was exactly what I wanted: a detail that could be fixed just like that.

'Can we go to Dr Palmer now?' I asked, thinking how nice it was to deal with as quick-moving a man as Dr Kelly.

But Dr Kelly, so brisk himself, was somewhat startled by my haste, and I realized with a sigh that *he* didn't have the pain.[17]

In recent years, historians have taken increasing interest in autopathographies written in letters and diaries.[18] Such writings can be especially insightful since they were written without thought of publication and hence unedited to strengthen or whitewash a point of view. They often reveal the importance attached to trust and faith in a particular doctor; as one patient wrote in a letter to a Dr Raine in 1887 saying that, since the doctor knew so much about his system and about his family and had prescribed for him oftener than any other since his marriage, he felt that the doctor could help him more than any other, even without seeing him.[19] Despite sharp differences in the practice of medicine between the past and present, analogous sentiments persist as already noted with Rachel Carson.

Patients' voices challenge doctors to reflect on whether they are hearing the many nuances in patients' questions and stories. After all, patients often feel they face 'professional listening', that is, the doctor listening only for information on symptoms that fit specific diagnoses; such listening tends to ignore or side-step a patient's worries as in *The Practice* quoted earlier in the chapter. At issue, too, is 'active' and 'passive' listening. In contrast to passive (perhaps listening with 'half an ear'), patients want active listening, which means a listener who concentrates on and understands everything that is being communicated, an approach facilitated by open-ended questions. It may even involve knowing when to be silent, when to respect a patient's silence, perhaps as they recollect painful events. Active listening can embrace many factors. For instance, it may be recognising that a patient's sense of time is different from that of a physician and that patients want to be allowed to talk for more than the '18 seconds', which has come to be viewed as the stereotypical time interval before a physician interrupts a patient with a question.[20] There is also the question of listening to families, including their silences. Ernest Hemingway's well-known short story, 'Indian Camp', leaves an indelible impression with the suicide of a husband who was ignored by the physician who performed an emergency caesarian section delivery of his child.[21]

Listening that hears and identifies concerns and worries, perhaps from intonations, may well help with 'healing' by finding meanings to an illness, connections for the patient and showing empathy (cf. Chapter 4 on healing).[22]

In some ways, professional listening is akin to the professional smile spotlighted by various authors. William Carlos Williams, in his 'The Use of Force', notices such a smile on a doctor as he tries to establish friendly communication with a child; its genuineness is questioned when he uses brute force to open the child's mouth.[23]

Medical responses

> I realized that the narrative skills I was learning in my English studies made me a better doctor. I could listen to what my patients tell me with a greater ability to follow the narrative thread of their story, to recognize the governing images and metaphors, to adopt the patients' or family members' point of view, to identify the sub-texts present in all stories, to interpret one story in the light of others told by the same teller.[24]

In the same discussion as this quote by Rita Charon, writing on 'Narrative Medicine', she makes clear how, for 13 years, she has worked to try to learn from patients in an organised fashion and that listening is the best way to learn about patients.[25]

The widespread public concerns over inappropriate communication have, as indicated, brought responses from the medical profession. Indeed, medical communication has developed as an academic area of study with the usual accoutrements of conferences, teaching materials and debates on how it should be taught.[26] Such a trend has sometimes registered with the popular press, as when a British newspaper reported on one medical communications conference under the heading: 'Doctors told how to talk to patients with cancer.'[27] One consultant stated: 'I regret for myself and my patient that I wasn't given this sort of opportunity before.' The reporter then added: 'Just under half of those who took part admitted that they had problems talking to patients of different ethnic and cultural backgrounds. A third found it hard to talk to the elderly, to children and to parents.' Further, an actor participating in the programme said: 'You did feel that some were ageist, sexist or racist, but in an unconscious form. There was not overt nastiness but it could be at the cost of communicating with the patients.'

By the 1990s, as noted, medical schools had begun to pay particular attention to interviewing and counselling skills, sometimes based on communication models that analyse word use and listener's responses and comprehension.[28] Moreover, more individual physicians, like Rita Charon, were beginning to appreciate that, depending on a patient's medical circumstances, listening and recording a patient's story about their illness might add much to a standard medical history that otherwise can be incomplete, not just in terms of the patient's humanity, but also that of the physician's.[29]

On the other hand, despite the growing awareness within medicine of the roles of narratives – and of the humanities in general – in contributing to reflection on communication skills, educational time is still more likely to be spent on specific 'difficult' (and important) areas such as how to deliver bad news. Many commentators, often patients, perceive that the general role of communicator is still fulfilled inadequately by many physicians, and regret that the early 2000s remain filled with 'horror stories' about bad medical communication.

In closing this chapter, we suggest that Epicetus' epigram could well be placed on the desk of every physician:

> Nature has given men one tongue, but two ears
> That we may hear others twice as much as we speak.

It can serve not only as a reminder about listening, but also of the related matters of appreciating, for instance, patients' time, the role of silence, and that the format of case history taking is designed for gathering quite specific information for the physician, and less about the overall psychological needs of the patient.

Endnotes

1 Cousins N (1983) *The Healing Heart: antidotes to panic and helplessness.* Norton, New York, pp. 132–3. It is noteworthy that the issue of medical errors noted by Cousins and constantly raised during the last decades of the twentieth century only achieved intensive examination by the professional organisations of medicine in the early 2000s with a sense that public lessons should be drawn from errors and mistakes.

2 For one discussion, still useful as an index of rising interest in the humanities, Ong LML, de Haes CJM, Hoos AM and Lammes FB (1995) Doctor–patient communication: a review of the literature. *Social Science and Medicine.* **40**: 903–18.

3 Davies R (1994) *The Cunning Man.* McLelland and Stewart, Toronto, pp. 216–17.

4 Holmes OW (1883) from 'The Young Practitioner' in his *Medical Essays 1842–1882.* Houghton Mifflin, Boston, p. 389.

5 The quote has been taken from a book of readings in which the editor offers comments on the novel, Furst LR (ed) (2000) *Medical Progress and Social Reality: a reader in nineteenth-century medicine and literature.* State University of New York, New York, p. 55.

6 It is relevant to add here that the definition of functional disease came to refer to conditions for which no *identifiable* pathology could be found. The concept created increasing difficulties for physicians and medical communication. In 1930, for example, a well-known American physician concerned with communication problems gently chastised colleagues with comments that some say are equally relevant today:

> In general hospital practice physicians are so busy with the critically sick, and in clinical teaching they are so concerned with training students in physical diagnosis and attempting to show them all types of organic disease, that they

do not pay as much attention as they should to the functional disorders. Many a student enters upon his career having hardly heard of them except in his course in psychiatry, and without the faintest conception of how large a part they will play in his future practice. At best, his method of treatment is apt to be a cheerful reassurance combined with a placebo. The successful diagnosis and treatment of these patients, however, depends almost wholly on the establishment of that intimate personal contact between physician and patient which forms the basis of private practice. Without this, it is quite impossible for the physician to get an idea of the problems and troubles that lie behind so many functional disorders. If students are to obtain any insight into this field of medicine, they must also be given opportunities to build up the same type of personal relationship with their patients.

(Peabody FW (1930) *Doctor and Patient: papers on the relationship of the physician to men and institutions*. The Macmillan Company, New York. Quote from pp. 45–6 from essay, 'The Care of the Patient', originally published in (1927) *Journal of the American Medical Association*, **88**: 877–82.)

7   Quote in Silverman ME, Murray TJ, and Bryan CS (2003) *The Quotable Osler*. American College of Physicians, Philadelphia, p. 56.
8   From a lecture on clinical medicine by Latham PM (1878) *The Collected Works of Dr PM Latham*, vol. 2. New Sydenham Society, London, pp. 29–30.
9   Letter to S Weir Mitchell, 6 January 1892. S Weir Mitchell Papers, Trent Collection, Duke University Medical Center.
10   All the postcards cards mentioned below in author's collection.
11   Sugarman J and Butters RR (1985) Understanding the patients: medical words the doctor may not know. *North Carolina Medical Journal*. **46**: 415–17.
12   It is of interest to add that even terms such as subcutaneous for labelling insulin preparations have been questioned: '"Subcutaneous" would not be understood by most [diabetic] patients.' (Gummerson I (2003) Do patients understand 'subcutaneous'. *Pharmaceutical Journal*. **270**: 50.)
13   Winchester S (1967) *The Practice*. Putnam's Sons, New York, pp. 30–2.
14   Poem quoted from Reynolds R and Stone J (eds) (1991) *On Doctoring: stories, poems, essays*. Simon and Schuster, New York, p. 187. Originally published in Myles J (1974) *To All Appearances*. University of Illinois Press, Chicago.
15   Pym B (1980) *A few green leaves*. In: Reynolds and Stone (1991) *On Doctoring*, p. 198.
16   See Aronson JK 'An Annotated Bibliography of Autopathographies,' www.clinpharm. ox.ac.uk/JKA/patientstale.html (accessed July 2004).
17   Gilfond D (1940) *I Go Horizontal*. The Vanguard Press, New York, p. 20.
18   Perhaps it should be added that the term 'autopathographies' is generally reserved for book length or other published accounts by patients; however, this is unnecessarily exclusive. One historian, Geoffrey Reaume, who in critiquing other historians for stereotyping those with mental illness, has used patients' voices to provide a humane view of mental illness: e.g. Reaume G (2000) *Remembrance of Patients Past: patient life at the Toronto Hospital for the Insane, 1870–1940*. Oxford University Press, Don Mills.
19   Letter written to Dr Raine by Eugena Coppedge from Cedar Rock, 22 March 1887. Quoted in Crellin JK (1993) *Tarheel Doctors and Patients*. Country Doctor Museum, Bailey, p. 16.
20   Beckman HB and Frankel RM (1984) The effect of physician behavior on the collection of data. *Annals of Internal Medicine*. **101**: 692–6 noted that in a mean time of 18 seconds physicians took control of a visit by asking increasingly specific, closed-ended questions that effectively halted the spontaneous flow of information from the patient. The figure continues to be widely quoted, sometimes with indications that, by 2004, physicians are spending longer times with patients.
21   The story is available in many publications/anthologies, e.g. Reynolds and Stone (1991) *On Doctoring*, pp. 139–42.

22   It may also mean that what some might view as 'category 2' symptoms are overlooked, symptoms that may point to an alternative diagnosis than is suggested by the cardinal symptoms.

23   For one of many discussions on the story, Bell BC (1985) Williams' 'The Use of Force', and first principles in medical ethics. *Literature and Medicine* **3**: 143–51.

24   Charon R, 'Narrative medicine': www.litsite.Alaska.edu/uaa/healing/medicine.html (accessed July 2004).

25   See also Delbanco T (2002) Listening and breaking down the walls. *Literature and Medicine*. **21**: 191–200.

26   As an example of a still important work, Cassell EJ (1976) *Talking with Patients*, vol. 1 *The Theory of Doctor–Patient Communication*. MIT Press, Cambridge and vol. 2 *Clinical Technique* (1985). This is an effective tool for classroom discussions. One of Cassell's examples of communication (vol. 2, pp. 164–7), which Cassell says meets all tests for effective communication – reducing uncertainty, providing a basis for action and strengthening the doctor–patient relationship – has been challenged. A socio-linguist, Bernard O'Dwyer (private communication) suggests that the particular example is, in fact, not effective communication, for a number of reasons. For instance, the doctor does not present his explanation in ordinary conversational context, and initially his approach might well intimidate. For instance, the use of the word skull, although understood by the patient, would have softer connotations if replaced with the word head. But of special interest is the patient's constant use of 'Mm-hm' in response to the physician's remarks. In conversations this often carries negative meanings such as 'I do not know what you are saying', 'Yes go on, I just want out of here', 'What does all this mean?', 'Am I seriously ill?'

27   *The Daily Telegraph*, 29 April 1998.

28   We might add that, apart from research carried out within the medical profession, socio-linguists – scholars who have a special competence in investigating the functions and consequences of a wide variety of social dialects – have noted the entrapment of physicians and patients in their separate languages. It is said that too often patients have to adjust to the physician's perspective and to learn 'doctor talk', where the opposite should be the case.

    As examples of the importance of plain language by physicians, one can cite court cases in British Columbia that have underscored the need to use simple language in communicating with patients. In one case, a dental surgeon was found liable for damages – resulting from the displacement of an impacted wisdom tooth – since he provided only printed information in technical language and, thereby, fell short of the requirements for informed consent. In another case, in January 1995, a judge from the British Columbia Court of Appeal said that an obstetrician/gynaecologist breached professional duty by not making clear how a bilateral tubal salpingectomy differed from tubal ligation. One issue is that, if patients do not understand, they may not ask the questions that trouble them. (See Gordon D (1996) MDs' failure to use plain language can lead to the courtroom. *Canadian Medical Association Journal*. **155**: 1152–3.)

29   It should be noted that there will always be issues of a physician's attitudes shaping their interpretation of a patient's account, indeed of the entire visit with a patient. Cf. Flood DH and Soricelli RL (1992) Development of the physician's narrative voice in the medical case history. *Literature and Medicine*. **11**: 64–83.

CHAPTER 4

Physician or healer?

It may come as a surprise that public expectations of physicians include the role of a healer. After all, physicians in general see themselves, as do many lay people, as healers.[1] Yet comments such as the following by a physician/professor of medical humanities command attention from physicians:

> As neurologists, my colleagues and I have complex objective measurements of the impact of a disease like MS [multiple sclerosis] on the nervous system. We can grade effects on various components of the neuraxis and on the person's mobility and function. However, when we have completed our neurological assessment, Kurtzke scales, function, and disability assessments, how well have we assessed the impact of the disease on this patient? Not very well, because we probably have not noted the impact of the disease on the person's self-image, relationships, hopes, and plans and its affects on the patient's personal and secret lives.[2]

Such comments are in tune with public opinions that healing must involve much more than attention to the physical aspects of a disease. Indeed, references to healing the mind and the spirit are common. This chapter draws attention to the meanings and expectations that the public attach to 'healing', a term that often overlaps with such others as holistic care. One consequence of the public voices is to ask physicians whether, in general, they offer healing as part of their treatment, and, if not, to what extent is it their responsibility to do so?

Healers: a diversity of images

What did Anatole Broyard mean when he said that he wanted his physician to be 'not only a talented physician, but a bit of a metaphysician, too'?[3] Although Broyard certainly wanted a doctor who was able to engage in conversation with him as an equal, seemingly he also wanted someone who could attend to, and perhaps heal, the mind. Countless people have expressed similar needs, not only in dealing with impending death, but also with a range of life's hurdles such as the death of a relative. At the same time, countless hopes exist, especially when conventional medicine has failed, that a healer can cure a physical ill, perhaps in unknown ways.

In the minds of the general public, healers are more likely to be lay people than physicians. Indeed, healers themselves may emphasise this for various reasons. Many use the term to avoid licensing regulations that protects the titles of various healthcare practitioners. They echo the non-medically qualified mental health therapist, in the British television movie *Murder in Mind* (1994), who felt the designation would help her to avoid prosecution for practising medicine without a licence. Healers have always come from diverse backgrounds. Countless numbers, commonly herbalists, work within a traditional (folkloric) medical system; they may practise with or without religious affiliation, sometimes as a result of receiving the 'gift' of healing (maybe because of being the seventh son of a seventh son). Their authority owes much to public confidence in the empirical tradition – experience accumulated over time – in contrast to a physician's knowledge, which is often characterised as being based more on theory and books. It is noteworthy that the complementary and alternative medicine movement of the second half of the twentieth century brought greater visibility to public confidence in empiricism; moreover, many of its practitioners emphasise (not always accurately) that a long history of usage demonstrates not only empirical evidence of safety and efficacy, but also of holistic care.

The authority of healers is often strengthened by their invocation of spiritual or magical forces; in fact these two aspects are interwoven in the practices of many healers. Spiritual care in western societies at the beginning of the twenty-first century often goes beyond time-honoured faith healing connected with particular religious followings – perhaps a miracle at Lourdes – to Interfaith and the New Age spirituality that draws, somewhat eclectically, on Eastern religions, on North American aboriginal spirituality and on the spirituality of other indigenous peoples. Indeed, a commonplace image of a healer is that of a shaman, medicine man or other native healer, an image reinforced by literature in many ways, such as novels set in Africa. For instance, Maria Thomas' *Antonia Saw the Oryx First* deals with the cultural and religious contexts of medicine in a story that centres around a Harvard-trained doctor returning to her African village and the daughter of a native healer who has also acquired the gift of healing.[4]

Hollywood is a fertile source of images of native healers. *Sunchaser* (1996), for example, noted in Chapter 2, tells of a terminally ill, half-Navajo 16-year-old searching for a medicine man. While in police custody, the teenager escapes and is able to hijack a physician to look after him medically while he searches. What had become something of a common indictment of conventional medicine – almost a cliché by 1996 – was spelled out in the film: 'Western medicine will forever regard symptoms of disease as simply errors to be corrected by drugs and surgery. You doctors will never do us any good until you wake up and learn not to poison. All healing comes from the divine within.'

Religious/educational writings are also forces in creating public images of healers. Healing stories such as the following, from the Catholic Health Association, about a Seminole boy in Florida have become common since the 1970s or so. One day, a young boy was brought to the clinic after falling from his bike and breaking an ankle. After his ankle was set and put in a cast, he was sent home. Later in the day, the physician talked to the village medicine man, who had visited the boy and enquired about the reason for breaking the ankle. After talking for some time, he asked the boy how he was getting along with his mother. 'The boy started to cry and explained that he and his mother weren't getting along well, in fact they weren't even speaking to each other. He picked up the boy and carried him to his mother, and they sat and talked together about the problem until it got resolved.' On being asked about how he came to ask the boy about his mother, the medicine man replied: 'for the Seminole, every part of the universe is represented by a part of the body, and the left ankle is the female.'[5]

A divide clearly exists between lay views of healers and healing – with its key components of empiricism and spirituality – and conventional medicine that is so often designated as 'scientific' or 'bio' medicine. It is a divide that sets the stage for criticism of the impersonality of much conventional care. Yet, as this chapter considers, perhaps the early 2000s is witnessing the building of a bridge across the divide with concepts of holism.

Holism and reductionism

> Every four days she washes his black body, beginning at the destroyed feet. She wets a washcloth and holding it above his ankles squeezes the water onto him, looking up as he murmurs, seeing his smile. Above the shins the burns are worst. Beyond purple. Bone.
>
> She has nursed him for months and she knows the body well, the penis sleeping like a sea horse, the thin tight hips. Hipbones of Christ, she thinks. He is her despairing saint. He lies flat on his back. No pillow, looking up at the foliage painted onto the ceiling, its canopy of branches, and above that blue sky.[6]

An opening scene in Michael Ondaatje's powerful novel, *The English Patient* (1992), conjures up many images as it sets a tone of mystery, drama and love. It also raises thoughts about the extraordinary nursing care, which continues to unfold in the story, for the man burnt beyond recognition. As readers learn about the nurse – who may also be viewed as a patient – questions about the nature of holistic care are raised. Like healing, the term 'holism' has a long history of various interpretations of its meanings; by the 1990s, however, it was generally understood as paying close attention to relationships between the body, mind and spirit.[7]

Complex reasons lie behind the growth of public interest in recent decades. One that artists commonly draw upon is a reaction to a sense of fragmentation in society and the uncertainty in what is so often described as our post-modern world. Cindy Sherman, for instance, in her paintings of what can be called patchwork bodies, suggests a fragmentary world. They have been described as 'monstrous pastiches, photographic collages of prosthetics, sex toys and dolls put together in combinations ... that make Frankenstein's monster positively benign.'[8] While some see Sherman's paintings as bizarre, they can be seen as symbolic of fragmented approaches to care. Laura Ferguson's sharply different 'Visible Skeleton Series' is another commentary. It is a visual enquiry into the artist's own curvature of her spine (scoliosis). It can be viewed as an attempt to understand her body by *integrating* accurate depictions of her spine with her feelings of self, a reaction to fragmentation. The results, she has said, were 'empowering, as if I were regaining a sense of ownership of my own body that had somehow been lost when my experience was "medicalized".'[9]

It is noteworthy that discussions on holism in the last two decades or so of the twentieth century, especially among those promoting complementary/alternative medicine, further fuelled the view, expressed by many medical humanities voices, that physicians commonly treat the disease and not the person. For instance, in the successful play *Wit*, by Margaret Edson, a resident physician sees a patient, Vivian, a formidable scholar of the work of John Donne, as a research subject rather than a patient.[10] Although such attitudes among physicians, now something of a cliché, have received justifiable criticism for overstatement, many see them as aptly describing what is seen as reductionism in medicine. This reductionism (with a long history, cf. Box 4.1), driven in large part by medical science and its demand to analyse parts, embraces tendencies to objectify or disembody physical aspects of the body from the vagaries of the mind.[11] Indeed, reductionism can be said to be a key concern about medical science. One poet, Bronwen Wallace, who succumbed to cancer at the age of 44, voices this in her poem, *Treatment*. She tells of a patient whom doctors talked of 'healing her flesh', while 'she told no one of her dream.' Her opening lines, with an economy of words, also give a sense of clinical detachment on the part of doctors when treatment becomes routine:

> For the doctors it seemed
> simple as an old war
> even the drug they used
> mechlorethamine
> a derivative
> of mustard gas dripped
> into her veins
> as she lay
> arms outstretched
> the chemical burning into her
> an older ritual
> given a new name
> demons to be exorcised
> a witch in need of cleansing[12]

Box 4.1   Reductionism and anatomy

Reductionism as an issue in medicine has had a long gestation period. It was certainly a thread in the seventeenth and eighteenth centuries. Then it owed much to seeing the body as a machine insulated from outside environmental influences. This is hinted at in an interesting by-way of medical humanities, namely changes in the nature of anatomical illustration, which suggest an increasing tendency to objectify the body. For instance, one can start with the muscle-men woodcuts in Vesalius' renowned 1543 anatomy text, *De Fabrica*. When the reverse images of the prints are placed in sequence, they reveal a continuous landscape as in the original artist's drawing that is tentatively attributed to Titian and his school. This continuous landscape cannot be discerned when viewing the muscle-men on each page as a result of the print making when each separate wood block became reversed. The point to be made is that this placing of anatomical figures in the context of nature was gradually expunged from anatomical texts over the next two centuries, just as anatomy ceased to raise questions about man's relationships with God as discussed in Chapter 8. For Vesalius: Cavanagh GST (1983) A New View of the Vesalian Landscape. *Medical History*. **27**: 77–9.

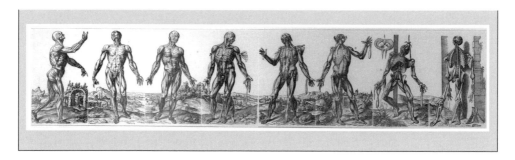

Many voices raise the same or similar concerns. The critically acclaimed novels of Walker Percy, for instance, prompt thoughts about the limitations of modern medicine in meeting the existential and spiritual needs so important to people in times of stress.[13] In his *The Second Coming* (1980), Will Barrett, the principal character, suffered from a strange collection of symptoms diagnosed as 'Hausmann's Syndrome' by the 'smart asshole' doctor from Duke University. The symptoms were 'depression, fugues, certain delusions, sexual dysfunction alternating between impotence and satyriasis, hypertension, and what he [Hausmann] called *wahnsinnige Sehnsucht* – [that is] inappropriate longing.'[14] However, treatment was said to be 'simple but pesky' in order to deal with an unstable pH. 'It means checking your pH every couple of hours and calibrating the medication accordingly.'[15]

Percy's concern with reductionism is clear in many places. Will Bennett's illness was not cured by chemistry alone. It was a love affair with Allison Huger, another person with a complex medical history, which brought about his final recovery. 'Our cases are similar,' said Allison, 'nowadays many psychosomatic conditions can be cured. I was reading in the *National Observer* at the A & P about the supremacy of mental attitude over physical conditions.'[16] In many ways, this was a retort to a remark made earlier by Will Barrett: 'A cool Carolina Salk rattling his test tubes at Duke had saved his life. How odd to be rescued, salvaged, converted by the hydrogen ion! A proton as simple as a billiard ball!'[17]

In another novel, *The Cunning Man*, appearing a few years later, Robertson Davies also spoke out for non-reductionist or holistic approaches. The main character, physician Jonathan Hullah, challenges readers to consider the reductionist mindsets of conventional medicine. After Hullah noted that a legend was growing up around him for using 'unconventional methods', he mused that 'there is nothing a professional group mistrusts so nervously as it does anything that appears unconventional, and that has not been thoroughly written up in the journals. It may be quackery. Worse still, it may be effective. And if it is both quackery and effective it is utterly hateful.' He goes on to say that he was not a quack. 'My dictionary says that a quack is somebody who professes a knowledge of which he is ignorant; but I profess nothing of the sort – I simply profess a knowledge of which a great many of my professional colleagues are ignorant.' Hullah saw himself as a humanist, although a friend called him a 'quodlibertarian physician, meaning that I mixed up all sorts of unlikely things to make a unity, choosing what I liked or what seemed best.'[18]

In his private correspondence, Davies was hardly flattering to physicians. In 1983, he commented that 'modern [Canadian] doctors have no god but the Canadian Medical Association.'[19] A few years later, in offering hope to a colleague diagnosed with cancer, he pointed out the counsel he seemingly used himself over time:

> Use three Physicians still
> First Doctor Quiet,
> Next Doctor Merryman
> and Doctor Diet.[20]

There is a clear sense that Davies, like Broyard, saw his ideal physician as a metaphysician; both, too, had in mind a humanist physician as a healer, rather than a lay person in the empirical/spiritual tradition. Hullah observes that he had 'heard people say that they could not be cured by a man who was obviously stupider than themselves. I myself have never responded to a doctor whom I thought illiterate, but that is sheer intellectual snobbery and of course I ought to be ashamed of it. But I'm not. However, I have never been able to do much for a patient I thoroughly disliked.'

Davies, like Walker Percy, also voiced the message that each person is to be treated individually – a way to understand connections between the body and the spirit. During World War II, when reading to wounded servicemen on Ward J, Davies' fictional physician observed that the reading 'would not restore an amputated leg, or bring back an errant girlfriend, but it would give a new look at those misfortunes and the new look was healing. I have been known to recommend another look at religion as a way to better health, or perhaps I should say well-being.'[21] Davies evidently saw the physician as the 'priest of our modern secular world',[22] and went on to say that he believed that 'there are as many stomachs, hearts, livers and lights as there are members of the human race, and that they should be treated individually to suit their special needs, whatever these might be. And those needs are not always found in the laboratory, but in the lay-confessional of the physician's consulting room.'[23]

Alongside the erudition of Percy and Davies, a myriad of popular books (some by physicians who extol mind–body interactions) and other facets of popular culture have also played on the theme of holism or mind–body connections in countless ways, from 'pop' psychology and New Age spiritualism to movies. In one example of the latter (*Body Parts*, 1991), limbs are transplanted from a multiple murderer to patients, along with, as it turns out, a predisposition to murder. In responding to the feelings of one patient with a transplant – 'I now have a murderer's blood in my blood' – the surgeon/scientist (a woman) said: 'scientifically speaking, the psychological make-up of the donor is irrelevant. It's *your* arm, not Fletcher's [the murderer].' Such a view was shattered by events. Although, appropriately, many see *Body Parts* as pure entertainment without a 'message', it can be seen as just one more thread in a web of disquiet in our popular culture about separating the mind and the body.

Some characteristics of healing

Both popular culture and academia have produced a vast range of articles that overlap as they deal with 'psychosocial care', 'healing', 'curing', 'wellness', 'holism', 'well-being' and 'spiritual care'. In general, all the articles point to at least three characteristics viewed as common, perhaps essential, components of healing that practitioners need to consider when evaluating their role in healing. The characteristics are empathy, helping to make connections and finding meanings.

1 *Empathy*. It is often suggested that one cannot learn how to be empathetic with a patient, commonly defined as 'I am you', or 'I could be you', or 'I can put myself in your shoes'. This contrasts with expressing sympathy that can be mere expressions of regret or sadness.

   Some suggest that true empathy only comes from the practitioner who has personal experiences of the same condition, or of other serious illness. This is not the situation for countless physicians. The question whether empathy can be learned is subject to much debate. Here we suggest that, for many people, empathy can be cultivated through what can be called 'informed imagination', or 'educated' or 'creative' imagination. In this, the eye of the visual artist, the pen of the creative writer, the illness narrative of a patient, the lens of the photographer can all provoke feelings and stir and educate imagination about what a particular patient needs.[24]

2 *Connections*. Making, or helping to make, connections for the sick person, whether it be through identifying 'spiritual' or transcendental links via formal religion, via the occult, life forces or nature, or by identifying support from family to support groups. Much of this may be seen as helping a person feel that they belong.

   There can be no doubt, as revealed in autopathographies, that it is especially important for patients to feel connected. Nowadays, with family members often separated by great distances, making or remaking family connections, especially among estranged members, can sometimes be difficult. The generally well-received film *Marvin's Room* (1996) that explores distant relatives, estranged relationships and the impact of chronic illness is one important resource in prompting thoughts about building and mending connections.

3 *Meanings*. Providing, or helping to provide, explanations or meanings to an illness. This might be merely providing a name to a condition: '"Is this throat of mine serious?" asks the patient. "No," says the doctor, "just pharyngitis." "Good," says the patient. The evil has lost its power.'[25] Or, 'meanings' can also serve as explanations or reasons for the suffering, perhaps due to religious or social transgressions. This can mean a physician's role is to understand their belief systems, and their cultural responses to illness and stress.[26]

   Anatole Broyard, when a patient, offered one challenging suggestion that can be viewed as a cross between finding a meaning and a coping mechanism: 'If the patient can feel that he has *earned* his illness – that his sickness represents the grand decadence that follows a great flowering – he may look upon his body as tourists look upon the great ruins of antiquity. Of course I'm offering these suggestions playfully, not so much as practical expedients but as experiments in thinking about medicine.'[27]

Other terms have been used to cover much of what has just been said. Compassion is one. Ralph Crawshaw's *Compassion's Way: a doctor's quest into the soul of medicine* – a collection of stories, reviews and vignettes written over many years – is a recommended journey in search of compassion that embraces empathy, connections and meaning. Crawshaw writes that his medical life has been a 'lifelong journey into the world of suffering, searching for meaning in suffering, [and] repeatedly finding it in companion's sharing.'[28]

Places of healing

An important topic in any consideration of healing can be the role of place, of the environment. While healers may work anywhere, sacred places and spaces have attracted much interest in recent times, prompted by popular fascination with native spirituality and ancient religious sites. These, often places where one is able to be close to nature or where generations have worshipped, contrast sharply with the modern hospital as Richard Selzer hints at more than once in his essays. In one, he stated strongly that he would not 'call a building *hospital* that did not have a fountain.'[29] On another occasion, he wrote that not long ago, operating rooms had windows that were a 'boon and a blessing in spite of the occasional fly that managed to strain through the screens and threaten our very sterility.' Selzer continues: 'the door to the next world sprang open. But for us who battled on, there was the benediction of the sky, the applause and reproach of thunder. A Divine consultation crackled in on the lightning! And at night, in Emergency, there was the pomp, the longevity of the stars to deflate a surgeon's ego.'[30] Selzer fears that, by bricking up windows, practitioners lose connections to the universe, to nature.

Analogous sentiments have been voiced in many ways, including by visual artists. For instance, Robert Pope's paintings of hospital life during his battle with cancer show the lonely and impersonal aspects of hospital treatment; evocative are scenes of looking through the windows of hospital rooms to nature on the outside (a sparrow on the top of a horse chestnut tree or at a mountain) or a church spire surmounted by a cross.[31]

The extent to which modern hospital architecture is designed to contribute to care of the mind, as has been the case in the past, is certainly problematic.[32] As noted in Chapter 2, functionalism came to be an overriding consideration in the twentieth century. A fascinating book that raises questions about healing environments and the changes that have occurred is Grace Goldin's *Work of Mercy: a picture history of hospitals* (1994), a book that closes with an account of the growing number of hospices in the 1980s and early '90s, and their role in healing at the end of life.[33] Not only does Goldin include photographs of a wide range of hospitals, but also paintings and prints. One painting is Johannes Beerblocks' *View of the Sick Ward of St John's Hospital* (1778). Although the large open ward accommodated many more patients than would ever be imagined today, each patient had some privacy in his or her own cubicle; moreover, the arches and hammered roof of the ward, and the aisles busy with the nursing nuns, priests and bishops soliciting gifts from wealthy citizens, offered connections to the community and spirituality that are generally absent from secular hospitals today. A clear sense exists that taking care of the soul, already with a long pedigree in the history of hospitals, was still a foremost consideration.[34]

Changes in healthcare environments are driven by many factors, not only by new diagnostic and treatment regimens, but also by changing emphases in patient care. Recently this has led to a return to concerns over the mind. For instance, beginning in 1996, Britain has seen the opening of a number of Maggie's Centres – innovative and inspiring cancer day-care centres.[35] The centres are in memory of Maggie Keswick Jencks, a cancer victim, whose experiences led her to write that most hospital environments seemingly say to patients: 'How you feel is unimportant. You are not of value.'[36] Of an eye-stopping centre in Dundee, renowned architect Frank Gehry has said: 'I hope the architecture won't override the purpose of the building, but complement it [cancer care] and take it to a higher plane of comfort and beauty.'[37] Explicit is the theme of the healing power of architecture.

A further consideration for healing, especially in life-threatening situations, is the extent to which patients need hope. Its role in healthcare has long been recognised though attitudes have changed in recent years. New hospitals are unlikely to include 'Hope' in their name as happened in the past.[38] That is not to say that hospitals, with all their modern technology, do not bring hope as they have in the past. Patients have often voiced this. In 1925, one penned the following message on a view postcard of the hospital:

> Dear 'Coz' – After 24 days in hospital & 2 operations [in 1925], I'm out again much the worse for wear but with the encouragement that they think they caused all my cancer to be disintegrated by this last radium which they used in a new way. Cutting down and putting many small radium needles in the tumour – If so I will be well. Have been too weak to do much writing. I'll write more fully soon. Love to all.[39]

What is especially striking is the far-reaching change in attitudes toward hope, as an integral part of treatment. From the 1960s onward diagnoses were no longer withheld from patients, one of the turning points in doctor–patient relationships. A survey carried out about the time of Rachel Carson's diagnosis of cancer (Chapter 2) asked cancer surgeons: 'What is your usual policy about telling patients? Tell? Don't Tell?' Ninety per cent who responded said that they would regularly withhold the truth. Only when patients refused to undergo treatment would doctors raise the stakes and introduce words and phrases calculated to signal the seriousness of the condition. The rationale was to protect the patient from despondency and loss of hope. Yet, Carson seems to be part of changing public attitudes. A Canadian survey at the time revealed what was becoming the norm, that two-thirds of women wanted to know the truth about their condition.[40] This view has prevailed, though not without angst among some physicians and patients about how to maintain hope while telling the patient the full truth about diagnosis and prognosis. One doctor with a serious illness, in perhaps suggesting that the whole truth should not always be told, spoke of the dilemma felt by many colleagues: 'As a patient I have learned that just as important as medical expertise and the proper use of new technology is the ability of the physician to show legitimate concern, to be there during the bad times, and to provide hope even to the incurable.'[41]

Responses

The widespread search for healing, physical and mental, often identified as holistic care, has, as indicated, impacted on institutions and individual practitioners in a number of ways. Here we add comments on the development of the healing arts movement and on some responses from the medical profession.

The healing arts

One of the roles for medical humanities is in patient care settings, either as medical therapy or as an approach to healing and wellness. Indeed much has been written on this in recent years, not only in terms of, say, art therapy, but also the role of the theatre, poetry, laughter (including clowning made public by the publications of, and movie about, Patch Adams[42]), movies for therapy,[43] music and more. Growing interest was evident in the 1950s, though what came to be called an arts for health movement only crystallised in the 1980s.[44] This not only contributes directly to patient care, but also offers new ways to explore healing.

One particular issue voiced amid the healing arts performers is that practitioners and patients often have different meanings of sickness. In the preface to a series of theatre monologues designed to prompt thoughts about what it means to be sick, actor/writer Leah Lewis writes that sickness is a difficult thing to write about for the theatre as the author is faced with the 'challenge to communicate truth and to avoid melodrama and indulgence.'[45] Sickness is not only the pain, but also, Lewis notes, loss of ownership of one's body as one is forced to give it over to strangers in order to achieve some level of comfort. She is concerned, too, that many people deny or reject sickness and the sick. 'We move away once we find out about an individual's ill health. We live in an active and demanding society. Sickness is not welcome among our everyday demands; there is no room for it. Sickness represents a stoppage. It represents weakness. It is not incorporated into what we've learned life to be.'

The theatre prods the imagination and feelings in ways different from novels and short stories, as does poetry, examples of which have already been used in this volume. A challenging book for healthcare practitioners, John Fox's *Poetic Medicine: the healing art of poem-making*, includes one physician's observation about ways it can contribute to finding meaning in ill-health: 'Our poetry allows us to remember that our integrity is not in our body, that despite our physical limitations, our suffering and our fears, there is something in us that is not touched, something shining. Our poetry is its voice. To hear that voice is to know the power to heal. To believe ... In times of crisis meaning is strength. But the deepest meaning is carried in the unconscious mind, whose language is the language of dreams, of symbols and archetypes. Poetry speaks this language, and helps us to hear meaning in illness.'[46] Poetry by patients is, in some cases, no more than narrative, the value of which we have already made clear. A physician's reading of a patient's poems and other writings can often provide insight into that person's condition. No doubt exists that the writings of the great twentieth-century poet Sylvia Plath challenge all those interested in diagnosing her mental suffering.[47]

Physicians' responses

We have noticed that the public do not necessarily view physicians as healers. However, an ambivalence also exists; after all, many physicians, with empathy for their patients and an appreciation of aspects of an illness related to the mind and spirituality, clearly fulfil the role of healer. Nevertheless, increasingly from the 1970s, physicians have been challenged from many directions (including from the complementary/alternative medicine movement) to be more proactive in paying attention to mind–body interactions in their care of patients. Some have responded.

As an illustration of change noticeable in the 1970s, Richard Selzer's 1976 story, 'The Surgeon as Priest', is noteworthy. It tells how an examination of a patient by Yeshi Dhonden, the personal physician to the Dalai Lama, gave the author new insight in connecting with patients and in healing.[48] After purification by bathing, fasting and prayer, the Tibetan physician examines the patient without knowing the western diagnosis:

> He steps to the bedside while the rest stand apart, watching. For a long time he gazes at the woman, favoring no part of her body with his eyes, but seeming to fix his glance at a place just above her supine form. I, too, study her. No physical sign nor obvious symptom gives a clue to the nature of her disease.
>
> At last he takes her hand, raising it in both of his own. Now he bends over the bed in a kind of crouching stance, his head drawn down into the collar of his robe. His eyes are closed as he feels for her pulse. In a moment he has found the spot, and for the next half hour he remains thus, suspended above the patient like some exotic golden bird with folded wings, holding the pulse of the woman beneath his fingers, cradling her hand in his. All the power of the man seems to have been drawn down into this one purpose. It is palpation of the pulse raised to the state of ritual. From the foot of the bed, where I stand, it is as though he and the patient have entered a special place of isolation of apartness, about which a vacancy hovers, and across which no violation is possible. After a moment the woman rests back upon her pillow. From time to time, she raises her head to look at the strange figure above her, then sinks back once more. I cannot see their hands joined in a correspondence that is exclusive, intimate, his fingertips receiving the voice of her sick body through the rhythm and throb she offers at her wrist. All at once I am envious – not of him, not of Yeshi Dhonden for his gift of beauty and holiness, but of her. I want to be held like that, touched so, *received*. And I know that I, who have palpated a hundred thousand pulses, have not felt a single one.

After a sensory examination of the urine, Yeshi Dhonden 'sets down the bowl and turns to leave. All this while, he has not uttered a single word. As he nears the door, the woman raises her head and calls out to him in a voice at once urgent and serene. "Thank you, doctor," she says, and touches with her other hand the place he had held on her wrist, as though to recapture something that had visited there.'

Afterwards, the staff physicians heard the Tibetan's diagnosis: 'winds coursing through the body of the woman, currents that break against barriers, eddying. These vortices are in her blood, he says. The last spendings of an imperfect heart. Between the chambers of her heart, long, long before she was born, a wind had come and blown open a deep gate that must never be opened. Through it charge the full waters of her river, as the mountain stream cascades in the springtime, battering, knocking loose the land, and flooding her breath.' This, probably to the surprise of many present, corresponded with the western diagnosis: a congenital interventricular septal defect of the heart with resultant heart failure.

Selzer comments: 'He is more than doctor. He is priest ... Now and then it happens, as I make my own rounds, that I hear the sounds of his voice, like an ancient Buddhist prayer, its meaning long since forgotten, only the music remaining. Then a jubilation possesses me, and I feel myself touched by something divine.'

Such challenges encouraged many physicians not only to explore spirituality in relation to health, but also to take an interest in the broad field of complementary/ alternative medicine, indeed to develop their own teaching about the mind and body. Surgeon Bernie Siegal is just one who became well known in the 1980s and '90s for his inspirational writings and talks that focused on visualisation and meditation in order for patients to give themselves 'live' and 'love' messages that can aid healing.[49] A number of physicians who have challenged conventional healthcare by becoming exponents of complementary/alternative medicine have chastised physician colleagues for not being healers.[50] They talk about the dehumanising atmosphere of medical schools (cf. also Chapter 8); thus L Dossey, for instance, has written that if medical schools are to produce healers, they must first stop destroying them. This, he believes, requires reducing or eliminating the many ways the medical school experience has become dehumanising.[51] And physician Andrew Weil has stated (1995):

> A great many practitioners of conventional medicine are very pessimistic about the possibility of healing. That pessimism has many roots, but certainly one of them is the fact that there is absolutely no teaching about healing in the medical curriculum today. It is not a focus of research. And I think this is the greatest defect in standard medicine today.[52]

Such critiques of medicine naturally frustrate physicians who have always pursued healing, or who recognise a relationship between the mind and body; after all, what is called psychosocial care or patient-centred care has been widely promoted in the profession for many years. Of course, doctors, all university educated, still have to face cultural mindsets that healing is associated with lay people, especially those who belong to an oral tradition and are nearer to the experiences of the past and to spirituality. This may challenge a physician to implement specific healing strategies such as to pursue a patient's narrative, to take a spiritual history,[53] and to respond to calls for prayer as therapy, if necessary to pray with patients in surgeries.[54]

Endnotes

1 Although the term 'healer' was not included in the original EFPO list, it is explicit in the original EFPO Working Papers noted in Chapter 1 in terms of public comments wanting humanist doctors and holistic care. The issue as to whether a physician can be described as a healer has been explored in academic texts. Analogies are often made between the shaman and modern medical practice, cf. May WE (1983) *The Physician's Covenant: images of the healer in medical ethics*. Westminster Press, Philadelphia.

2 Murray TJ (1995) Healing when there is no cure. *Humane Medicine*. **11**: 94–5.

3 'The patient examines the doctor', in Broyard A (1992) *Intoxicated by My Illness*. Clarkson Potter, New York, p. 40.

4 Thomas M (1987) *Antonia Saw the Oryx First*. Soho, New York.

5 *Spirituality and Health: what's good for the soul can be good for the body too.* (1996) Catholic Health Association of Canada, Ottawa, pp. 19–20.

6 Ondaatje M (1992) *The English Patient*. Vintage Books, Toronto, pp. 3–4.

7 See, for instance, Lawrence C and Weisz G (eds) (1998) *Greater than the Parts: holism in biomedicine, 1920–1950*. Oxford University Press, New York.

8 Quoted in Crellin JK (2000) Fragmentation and holism. *MunMed*. **4**: 3. (Faculty of Medicine, Memorial University of Newfoundland.)

9 Ferguson L (2004) 'The visible skeleton series': artist's introduction. *Perspectives in Biology and Medicine*. **47**: 165–8.

10 Edson M (1999) *Wit*. Faber & Faber, New York.
11 For criticism from a significant exponent of more holism in healthcare, Cousins N (1979) *Anatomy of an Illness as Perceived by the Patient: reflections on healing and regeneration*. Norton, New York, pp. 109–10. Chapter on holistic health and healing.
12 Wallace B (1983) *Signs of the Former Tenant*. Oberon, Ottawa, p. 90.
13 For overview and various perspectives, see papers in Elliott C and Lantos J (eds) (1999) *The Last Physician: Walker Percy and the moral life of medicine*. Duke University Press, Durham.
14 Percy W (1980) *The Second Coming*. Farrar Strauss Giroux, New York, pp. 301–2. For full discussion, Majeres KD (2002) The Doctor and the 'Delta Factor': Walter Percy and the dilemma of modern medicine. *Perspectives in Biology and Medicine*. **45**: 579–92.
15 *The Second Coming* (1980), p. 303.
16 Ibid., p. 344.
17 Ibid., pp. 306–7.
18 Davies R (1994) *The Cunning Man*. McClelland and Stewart, Toronto, p. 246.
19 Grant JS (ed) (1999) *Robertson Davies. For Your Eye Alone. Letters 1976–1995*. McClelland and Stewart, Toronto, p. 113.
20 Ibid., p. 264; also the same verse to another correspondent, p. 165.
21 Ibid., p. 248.
22 Ibid., p. 217.
23 Ibid., p. 247.
24 This is underscored in writings on empathy such as Spiro HM, Curnen MGM, Peschel E and St James D (1993) *Empathy and the Practice of Medicine: beyond pills and the scalpel*. Yale University Press, New Haven.
25 O'Donnell M (1995) The toxic effect of language on medicine. *Journal of the Royal College of Physicians of London*. **29**: 525–9.
26 This is not the place to explore belief systems here; however, insofar as medical humanities is concerned with individuals, it is important to understand differences between the concepts of conventional medicine and lay beliefs of health and disease. The former can be readily characterised by:

    1 a strong preference for action
    2 a belief that humankind can and should dominate nature
    3 a belief that individuals can and should improve themselves by their own efforts
    4 a belief in the authority of objective experience.

    Lay health belief systems, on the other hand, are often a complex of integrated and rational beliefs linked to notions of balance within the body or cleansing the body. This may be supported by:

    1 a belief that health is a product of balance and harmony that may extend to community and family involvement
    2 a belief that individuals cannot and should not control nature
    3 a belief in the authority of subjective experience.

    Apart from ideas of supernatural or metaphysical causation of disease, other concepts of causation found in lay health belief systems include:

    1 theories of degeneration in which illness follows the running down of the body
    2 mechanical theories in which illness is the outcome of blockages or damage to bodily structure
    3 theories of invasion which includes germ theory and other material intrusions.

    For illustrations of many current issues, especially in multicultural settings, see case history in O'Connor BB (1995) *Healing Traditions: alternative medicine and the health professions*. University of Pennsylvania Press, Philadelphia, pp. 82–105. The case illustrates the complexity of religious beliefs to be found in increasingly multicultural societies.

27 Broyard (1992) *Intoxicated by my Illness*, p. 48

28 Crawshaw R (2002) *Compassion's Way: a doctor's quest into the soul of medicine*. Medi-Ed Press, Bloomington, p. 36.

29 Selzer R (1992) *Down from Troy: a doctor comes of age*. William Morrow, New York, p. 92.

30 Selzer R (1979) An Absence of Windows. In his *Confessions of a Knife*. Simon and Schuster, New York, pp. 15 and 21.

31 Pictures included in Pope R (1990) *Illness and Healing: images of cancer*. Lancelot Press, Hantsport.

32 The history of hospitals is now vast, but for some introduction concerning hospitals as therapy, as distinct from medicine for the soul (see below), Edginton B (1994) The well-ordered body: the quest for sanity through nineteenth-century architecture. *Canadian Bulletin of Medical History*. **11**: 375–86; questions are also raised in Thompson JD and Golden G (1975) *The Hospital: a social and architectural history*. Yale University, New Haven Press.

33 Goldin G (1994) *Work of Mercy: a picture history of hospitals*. Associated Medical Services/ Boston Mills Press, Toronto. For hospice movement, Du Boulay S (1984) *Cicely Saunders, Founder of the Modern Hospice Movement*. Hodder and Stoughton, London.

34 For an introduction to the theme, Henderson J (2001) Healing the body and saving the soul: hospitals in renaissance Florence. *Renaissance Studies*. **15**: 188–216.

35 Glancey J (2003) Cancer clinic designed to lift the spirits. *Guardian Weekly*. 16–22 October, p. 16.

36 Ibid.

37 www.arcspace.com/architects/gehry/maggies (accessed July 2004).

38 Various commentators focus on lack of trust in hospitals, for instance Bogdanich W (1991) *The Great White Lie: how America's hospitals betray our trust and endanger our lives*. Simon and Schuster, New York.

39 Message mailed in 1925 on a postcard (author's collection) showing a view of the hospital; radium therapy, arising from the celebrated studies of Marie Curie (1867–1934), was a popular cancer treatment for many years. Hope from the new medicine, however, did not mean that alternatives were not being tried, either within conventional medicine or the many so-called 'quack' cures.

40 Leopold E (1999) *A Darker Ribbon: breast cancer, women and their doctors*. Beacon Press, Boston, pp. 122–3.

41 Aoun H (1992) From the eye of the storm, with the eyes of a physician. *Annals of Internal Medicine*. **116**: 335–8.

42 Cf. Adams P with Mylander M (1998) *Gesundheit*. Healing Arts Press, Rochester; Adams P (1998) *House Calls: how we can heal the world one visit at a time*. Robert D Reed, San Francisco.

43 An interesting website is Christian Spotlight that includes 'Movies for Therapy'. 'Movies can be more than entertainment; they can be therapeutic – helping people see themselves, others, or issues in a new light. They can open up productive dialogue.' See: www.Christiananswers.net/spotlight/movies/therapy.html (accessed December 2003).

44 J Palmer, 'An introduction to the Arts for Health movement, or how the arts sneaked in on the medical model': www.communityarts.net/readingroom/archive/intro-health. php (accessed July 2004). Healing environments for patients, visitors and staff of hospitals, hospices and other health centres are being encouraged by 'healing gardens, paintings in patients' rooms, live music in lobbies and on patients' units, and art that helps people find their way through large and confusing buildings. Its impact is seen as rejuvenation, seen to range from helping to rejuvenate staff to specific outcomes of patient care.'

45 Notes provided for class performances of *Spelunking* (unpublished) to medical students in the Faculty of Medicine, Memorial University of Newfoundland.

46 Fox J (1997) *Poetic Medicine: the healing art of poem-making*. Jeremy P Tarcher/Putnam, New York, pp. xiii-xiv. (Preface by physician Rachel Remen.)

47 Cf. just one recent article, Cooper B (2003) Sylvia Plath and the depression continuum. *Journal of the Royal Society of Medicine*. **96**: 296–301.

48 Selzer R (1976) The surgeon as priest. In his *Mortal Lessons: notes on the art of surgery*. Simon and Schuster, New York, pp. 33–6. Note also the writings of physician, G Epstein,

who became generally well known for his emphasis on imagery, e.g. his (1994) *Healing Into Immortality: a new spiritual medicine of healing stories and imagery.* Bantam Books, New York.

49 Various websites attest to the interest in Bernie Siegel's teaching, e.g. www.brian weiss.com/kindred/siegel.htm (accessed July 2004).

50 In turn, such physician promoters are often chastised for being unscientific or indiscriminately selecting from the literature – the same criticism that extends to physician critics of other aspects of medicine. Cf. Morrison AR (2002) Perverting medical history in the service of 'animal rights'. *Perspectives in Biology and Medicine.* **45**: 606–19.

51 Dossey L (1995) Whatever happened to healers? *Alternative Therapies in Health and Medicine.* **1** (5): 6–13.

52 Weil A (1995) The body's healing systems. The future of medical education. *Alternative and Complementary Therapies.* **1** (5): 305–31.

53 For relevant discussion: Maugans TA (1996) The SPIRITual History. *Archives of Family Medicine.* **5** (1): 11–16. The author suggests the following pnemonic for case history taking: **S** – Spiritual Belief System; **P** – Personal Spirituality; **I** – Integration and Involvement in a Spiritual Community; **R** – Ritualised Practices and Restrictions; **I** – Implications for Medical Care; **T** – Terminal Events Planning (Advance Directives). A 1999 US survey reported that almost two-thirds would want a doctor to ask whether they had spiritual/religious beliefs that would influence their medical decisions if they became gravely ill. See Mansfield CJ, Mitchell J and King DE (2002) The doctor as God's mechanic? Beliefs in the Southeastern United States. *Social Science and Medicine.* **54**: 399–409. It is noted that in rural North Carolina 80 per cent of respondents believe that God acts through physicians to cure illness.

54 The literature on spirituality/religion in relation to healthcare is now vast, including ethical issues. For one useful introduction, Cohen CB, Wheeler SE, Scott DA *et al.* (2000) Prayer as therapy: a challenge to both religious belief and professional ethics. *Hastings Center Report.* May–June: 40–7. Magaletta PR, Duckro PN and Staten SF (1997) Prayer in office practice: on the threshold of integration. *Journal of Family Practice.* **44**: 254–5.

CHAPTER 5

Role as a scientist: questions about integrity

Alongside public concerns over the humanistic side of healthcare, expectations exist that physicians fulfil the role of a scientist, at least as a scientist-scholar.[1] However, it has to be asked what exactly does the public mean by wanting the physician to possess the role of scientist? It is, after all, unclear just how many people want their *personal* physician to be a 'medical scientist', rather than just being up to date on medical science. Attitudes towards one's personal physician – which can vary according to the severity of the illness – have long reflected or fallen between two well-staked-out, contrasting positions. One position is unquestioned acceptance that medical scientists are central to medicine, which must be practised on the basis of science. This embraces expectations that, in time, medical science will fill gaps in our current knowledge of diseases and cures. The second position, one always hovering in popular culture, questions the motives and integrity of medical scientists, who are often stereotyped as cold and aloof, and ready to 'experiment' on patients.[2]

The latter position is bolstered from various directions. One is the long-standing and continuing attacks on 'heartless scientists' from the antivivisection movement. In the 1970s and '80s such attacks became increasingly conspicuous, often with campaigns to protect animal rights, and arguments that alternative means of testing pharmacologically active preparations needed to be found. Media accounts such as the following that, at face value, challenged the moral probity of science tended to inflame public attitudes:

> Robert White, a professor of neurosurgery in Cleveland, has success-fully transplanted heads on monkeys. Because nerve fibres could not be reattached, the bodies were paralyzed but capable of pumping blood to their new heads, which were conscious, according to a news report. The animals kept up a cycle of waking and sleeping, ate and drank, followed laboratory staff with their eyes and could react to noises. They survived for a week.[3]

This chapter, in elaborating on the spectrum of public attitudes to medical science, notices various images of scientists and their role in experimentation. In so doing, questions arise about the extent to which the negative images cast a shadow over the entire medical profession, and how much they contribute to public mistrust of medical science.[4]

From heroic images to 'experimenting' on patients

Innumerable positive public images of medical science support the view that it is central to the advance of and the authority of medicine. The influence of popular writings on 'heroes' such as Louis Pasteur, Paul Ehrlich, Alexander Fleming and other international icons to be found in medical halls of fame can hardly be overestimated.[5] Artists, too, have been influential. In Philadelphia, what can be viewed as the ennobling of surgery emerged with the giant canvas paintings by Thomas Eatkins: 'The Gross Clinic' (1875) and 'The Agnew Clinic' (1889). It has been said that while the pictures are in the realist tradition that portrays the dignity and even the heroism of daily work and labour, by taking the public into the inner sanctum of surgery, so to speak, they point up the honour and prestige of surgery that was witnessing many advances at the time.[6]

Other heroic vignettes are woven into public thinking from time to time, such as self-experimentation (autoexperimentation) or experimenting on one's own family. An intriguing book, *Who Goes First? The Story of Self-Experimentation in Medicine*, lists innumerable names ranging from John Hunter, the celebrated eighteenth-century surgeon who may well have contracted gonorrhoea and syphilis as a result of self-inoculation, to members of the US Yellow Fever Commission (1900); the latter's mission – to discover whether the disease was transmitted by mosquito bites – led to the death of Jesse Lazear, one of the investigators acting as a guinea pig for mosquito bites.[7]

Popular culture has, at times, been accepting of heroic experiments on patients – fact and fiction – at least when there was a positive outcome for the patient. One example appears in the movie *Doctor Kildare's Strange Case* (1940) in which Kildare, without the necessary clinical experience or administrative permission, administers the relatively new insulin shock treatment to a deranged man and thereby brings him back to sanity. Perhaps such images encourage the acceptance of new non-fictional procedures even when they are initially disappointing, as in heart transplantation. Many accept that there are necessary steps on the road to ultimate heroic triumph. The latter has been extolled many times in prose and verse; Miroslav Holub's long poem, 'Heart Transplant', closes:

> and when the heart begins to beat
> and the curves jump
> like synthetic sheep
> on the green screen,
> it's like a model of a battlefield
> where Life and Spirit
> have been fighting
>
> and both have won.[8]

Contrasting with heroic medical experiments are frequent questions about excessive laboratory testing of patients, including experimentation without patients' consent ('experimentees' as they have been labelled). Indeed this identifiable thread throughout the twentieth century has fostered much public uncertainty and ambivalence. Uneasy relationships between physicians were evident in the early decades of the twentieth century when colleagues critiqued each other for over-reliance on laboratory-based data in their practices. Esteemed British physician Sir James Mackenzie, for instance, wrote (1918) that 'laboratory training *unfits* a man for his work as a physician' since it accustoms him to mechanistic ways of thinking. Too much science, too much specialisation, too many hours amid the test tubes might produce a fragmentation of the mind not conducive to healing.[9] Patients could be seen as walking organs and diseases, not persons. By 1928, a leader in the American medical profession commented: 'it is rather fashionable to say that the modern physician has become "too scientific".'[10]

Around the same time – the 1920s and '30s – questions about the ethics of medical science were brought before the public with two acclaimed, now classic, novels. Best sellers from their release, both, along with powerful movie versions, have become significant voices summarising persistent questions about medical science and its motivations. The earliest, *Arrowsmith* (1925) by Sinclair Lewis, follows the principal character, Dr Martin Arrowsmith, from general practitioner to research scientist, from his breakthrough discovery of a treatment for the plague to disillusionment with the bureacracy of science, and finally to find integrity in private scientific research.

A key issue – Arrowsmith's dilemma in being both physician and scientist – arose from the need for a randomised trial of his bacteriophage treatment on an island in the West Indies; the trial was to deprive half the population of the new 'life-saving' treatment. As Arrowsmith's teacher and role model, Max Gottlieb, said: 'You must not be just a good doctor at St Hubert. You must pity, oh, so much the generation after generation yet to come that you can't let yourself indulge in pity for the men you will see dying.'[11] However, on the death of his wife from the outbreak, Arrowsmith breaks down, drinks heavily, shouts 'damn experimentation', and becomes a 'traitor' to science by giving the 'phage to everyone who asked.'[12] Long after publication, the book continues to offer relevant 'messages'. In 2002, a physician/historian wrote in an article, 'Prescribing Arrowsmith': 'as the ties between medical scientists and the biotechnology industry become increasingly intertwined, the doctor in me wished he could prescribe a page or two of *Arrowsmith* each day to his more profit-driven colleagues. Perhaps "Dr Lewis" could restore some health to the ailing condition of scientific idealism.'[13]

In the second book, *The Citadel* (1937) by novelist–physician AJ Cronin, a physician's loss of idealism has parallels to *Arrowsmith*. Dr Manson's youthful research in his very first practice, in which he identified the role of 'silicosis' among miners, was cut short when the latter, suspicious of his home laboratory with its guinea pigs, drew the wrath of antivivisectionists. Subsequently, Manson's ideals for improving medicine are vanquished when, in need of income, he moves into the role of 'society' doctor and becomes involved with unnecessary treatment and fee-splitting among doctors. His medical idealism is reawakened following the death of a patient. Subsequently, his successful treatment of another patient, in association with an unlicensed 'quack', led to disciplinary charges by the licensing authority, the General Medical Council. The ending of the film version of *The Citadel* is memorable for Manson's fiery defence, before the Council's disciplinary hearings, of his collaboration with the unlicensed practitioner: 'What if we [the medical profession] go on trying to make out that everything is right inside the profession and everything wrong outside, it will be the death of scientific progress.' Of special interest, too, is a statement at the beginning of the movie – a response linked to the criticism of the novel by the medical profession:

> This motion picture is a story of individual characterisations and is in no way intended as a reflection of the Great Medical Profession which has done so much toward beating back those forces of nature that retard the physical progress of the human race.

Popular critiques of the 'Great Medical Profession', at least in terms of what is seen as exclusive attention to science, have sharpened dramatically in recent decades. Today's new legal requirements of adequately informed consent by patients merely underscores throw-away lines in popular culture about experimenting on patients. In the movie *K-PAX* (2001), for instance, one psychiatrist responds to another about a possible treatment for a patient with the remark: 'What! Experiment on him before we have a diagnosis?' In one sense, public concerns with science are a protest against imperial attitudes of scientists perceived as impersonal, often as a consequence of a research or reductive mindset. This is an underlying theme in the 'true' story told in the movie *Lorenzo's Oil* (1992). Augusto Odone – the father of a young son, Lorenzo, with adrenoleukodystrophy, a fatty acid disorder that produces demyelination of the nerves – proclaims at an open meeting of a support group: 'Our children seem to be at the service of medical science. We thought medical science was the servant of suffering children.' Lorenzo's parents then begin their own excursion into science to find a treatment for their son; ultimately, they developed a mixture of oleic and erucic acids (Lorenzo's oil) that, theoretically at least, could stem the demyelination. The somewhat negative, stonewalling image of physicians in the movie – despite the presence of avuncular, fatherly actor Peter Ustinov as the key physician–researcher – has perhaps been countered in recent years by the view that Lorenzo's oil is not a cure, even if it slows the development of symptoms. Despite concerns about the accuracy of the film in recounting the 'real' story, one physician's comments on the film are salutary. 'Although overlong and overdone, the film raises important issues by portraying attitudes of lay people that physicians and researchers ignore at their peril.'[14]

From time to time, small but cumulatively significant voices from popular culture also provoke unsettling thoughts about research ethics. An evocative postcard (2000), for example, includes the following information alongside a physician undertaking a lung biopsy. In 1996, a 19-year-old University of Rochester student, Nicole Wan, volunteered for a routine lung cell removal procedure for which she was to be paid $150. She suffered cardiac arrest a few hours after she left the research unit due to a fatal dose of lidocaine, and did not recover. The card's editorial comment is that 'if you get an adverse reaction they kick you out of the study ... so you tend to downplay things like headaches and mild nausea.'[15]

Even more provocative is the voice of artist Christine Borland that questions the use of human tissue without the person's consent. For instance, her installation, *Hela, Hot 2001*, challenges viewers to contemplate Henrietta Laks, who died of cancer in the 1950s; her cells, taken for diagnostic purposes, are now, without her permission, widely used in medical research (HeLa cells) because of their ability to divide rapidly.[16]

Lastly, we notice again medical thrillers (Chapter 2, Box 2.2) that often centre plots around black sheep in the medical profession. For example, in Michael

Palmer's *Miracle Cure* (1997), the villain physicians are part of the science-based pharmaceutical industry. A new 'miracle' drug is about to be marketed for athereosclerotic arterial disease, when the whistle-blower – a physician with principles – determines that experiments and data are faked to hide evidence of dangerous side-effects. The moral fallibility and financial greed of physicians, at least the black sheep, are part of the central plot. All this adds to frequent media reports about the way the pharmaceutical industry wields its commercial power to fund research on drugs (thus opening the door to inherent biases among researchers) and to persuade physicians to use particular brands.[17]

Technology

Threading throughout the hovering public concerns already raised are culturally entrenched fears of technology and science. Ever present images, from Frankenstein to genetically modified organisms, prompt thoughts whether much of the research is taking society on a downward path to destruction.

One of the most enduring images – often a metaphor for the fears of out-of-control science – is undoubtedly Frankenstein, created in Mary Shelley's 1818 novel, *Frankenstein or The Modern Prometheus*. Young Viktor Frankenstein, a brilliant student, discovered how to create life from dead body parts. Thus was created the 'monster' that, over time, has gone through countless reincarnations and adaptations in stories, plays, prints and movies. An 'industry' of commentators generally interpret the influence and persistence of the monster as raising fears and doubts about science and technology and of its irresponsible use. The monster, when depicted in the 1994 movie version as an intelligent 'human', reminded audiences of ethical issues in saying to Frankenstein: 'Did you ever think of the consequence of your actions?'[18]

In contrast to the life force that brings Frankensteinian monsters alive, cyborgs are artificially enhanced human beings. They contrast with androids (totally mechanical, even if human in appearance), although the borderline can be indistinct as in the popular *Terminator* and *Robocop* movies.[19] Along with public fascination with science fiction's forecasts of the future are its foreboding messages about tampering with genetic make-up, a theme often coupled with images of mad scientists. For instance, in the 1996 movie *The Island of Doctor Moreau* – based on HG Wells' novel of the same title (1896), albeit more loosely than two earlier film versions (1933 and 1977) – Moreau, as a mad scientist, upsets the balance of nature with genetic experiments that splice animal and human DNA, and turns a South Sea island heaven into hell when the beast-men band together to take control.

Although science fiction, especially that which goes beyond the bounds of imagination, is not universally popular, it has a major cultural presence as it mixes hope and optimism with fears for the future of the human race. Hopes and optimism, for example, that mechanical joints will soon be mobilised by paralysed people through their thought processes, and that small mechanical hearts will come into everyday use. On the other hand, there are fears that technology could ultimately undermine society and turn it into scenarios such as depicted in the well-respected science fiction story, *Bladerunner* (1974).[20] Written by physician Alan Nourse, the story centres on an overpopulated world where medical attention is either received at great price (coercive sterilisation) or through underground doctors serviced by 'bladerunners', who deliver surgical instruments to outlaw doctors who cannot obtain them legally.

The fears of, or at least ambivalence towards, science/technology that are embedded in popular culture also draw on mixed promotional messages from the healthcare professions and from industry. For instance, a large advertisement from a Canadian chain of pharmacies for 'Life Brand Sparkling Water Beverage Mixed Berry' featured a bottle of the water in front of two white-coated men under the caption: 'Made with no caffeine, sodium or scientists.'[21] The fears, too, reflect the considered opinions of thoughtful academics who ask searching questions about technology and its continual preoccupation with standardisation and efficiency that takes on a life of its own; one question is whether humanity will become technology's slave.[22]

Many physicians also express concerns. Few current voices are more effective than Rafael Campo in asking whether physicians have become too dependent on technology – a current rendering of concerns about over-dependence on laboratory medicine already raised, as noted, by the beginning of the 1900s. For example, in his short poem 'Technology and Medicine', Campo writes of his eyes as microscopes and cathode X-ray tubes, his hands as hypodermic needles, and so on.[23] In his own observations on the poem he indicates that it expresses feelings he sometimes has with patients. During medical school and residency he felt he was 'becoming machine-like in my interactions' with patients. 'Whereas I think in many ways technology can, when used properly, help us to form human connections and to nurture those connections. Oftentimes I think particularly some of the machines we use in medicine can really put obstacles between us and separate us in ways that are problematic for me. For example, looking at an X-ray of a patient without for a moment thinking of what that X-ray really shows in terms of their bodies. I think oftentimes when I'm looking at CAT-scans and interpreting the findings I see there that I'm looking through the patient. I'm not seeing what they're really thinking.'

Another influential physician's voice is Richard Selzer. Noteworthy is his 'The Virgin and the Petri Dish', published shortly after the birth (1978) of the first 'test tube' baby, Louise Brown, conceived by *in vitro* fertilisation.[24] It was a time of much public disquiet and uncertainty – with talk of monstrous babies, eugenics and irresponsible reproductive engineering – that heralded ongoing vigorous debates over the increasing invasiveness of techniques of reproductive technology. Nothing, as Selzer makes clear, could be more different from the virgin birth ('hallowed beyond all other conceptions') than artificial reproduction using a petri dish (not, as Selzer points out, a test tube). Selzer employs evocative word pictures. On conventional fertilisation he wrote: 'By the soft undulation of membranes and the waving of a million tiny paddles, the Fallopian tube propels the egg the whole length of its canal until, at last, having brought the egg to the horn of the uterus, the little pearl of great price is relinquished. Like an enclosed garden in which the rarest of plants is to be grown, the womb has been raked clean of all weeds and debris, and made ready to receive the egg.' Although Selzer appreciates the skill and technology of petri dish fertilisation, and recognises its place, he leads readers to ask where such new technology is taking us: 'And what of the memories past to which each of us is heir? If we are to believe the poets, philosophers and psychoanalysts, our embryonic lives, though unremembered, are there to be drawn upon in moments of inspiration or anguish.'

Today's readers of Selzer's essay point out that public anxiety over *in vitro* fertilisation has declined in the face of the countless thousands of resultant births since 1978, and, therefore, has become a 'norm' within medicine. Yet issues persist, such as how far should life be medicalised? How does society and medicine establish scientific norms? Further, Selzer's reference to the virgin birth is a reminder of the long-standing difficult relationships between formal religion and science over time. Although, for the most part, religion–science controversies nowadays are far removed from the intensity that once surrounded Darwin's theory of evolution, they still prompt debate on the reductionism and the arrogance of science. The movie *Agnes of God* (1985) explores such matters. A newborn child is found dead in a convent. The baby's mother, and possibly murderer, Sister Agnes is other-worldly and amnesic about the birth. A female psychiatrist assigned to the case – a chain-smoking, agnostic representative of rational science, hardly an endearing character – cannot consider any explanation for the situation other than murder, certainly not a virgin birth.

Scientific fraud

> When Krauss couldn't repeat my experiment, I got scared [writes a graduate student]. I thought it was due to my sloppy notes … that I'd missed something important. When we repeated the experiment in Cantor's lab, I tried to be extra careful. But after a while, IC's [my supervisor, Professor Cantor] continuous looking over my shoulder and checking every detail against the notebook got me real edgy. The day before we were supposed to be finished – a Sunday – I had just gone home, when suddenly I realized that earlier in the day I had added too little kinase.

The graduate student in Carl Djerassi's novel, *Cantor's Dilemma* (1989), continues to relate that he returned to the lab, without informing his supervisor, and added some more enzyme. 'I don't think this was real fudging. I calculated how much kinase I had missed earlier and then just made up for it. I know I should've told IC, but I didn't have it in me. First my sloppy notebook, and then that stupid mistake.'[25]

Arguably, stories of scientific fraud may be the most potent factor casting shadows over the integrity of medical science. Additional to the already mentioned world of medical thrillers, *Cantor's Dilemma* is a realistic view of the competitive world of scientific research. Djerassi, an internationally renowned scientist, does not deal with outright fraud – not the black-and-white issues as in many thrillers; instead he 'maps out much greyer territory into which we scientists, deliberately or inadvertently, sometimes stray.'[26]

Djerassi's interest in scientific integrity is also reflected in his later novels that he describes as being in the genre of 'science in fiction'; in this, unlike science fiction, all the science 'does or could exist.'[27] The novels give a sense as to how subtle biases can enter into scientific research – an issue that has come to the fore in recent years.[28] In fact deliberate fraud, often stranger than fiction, was already making headlines when *Cantor's Dilemma* first appeared. The book *Fraud and Misconduct in Medical Research* sees 1974 as a real starting point of concern over piracy, plagiarism and forgery due to publicity surrounding William Summerlin and his use of the felt-tip pen to fake a successful skin transplant from a black to white mouse.[29] More bizarre than Summerlin's felt-tip pen is a peer-reviewed paper published in the *British Journal of Obstetrics and Gynaecology* in 1997 that turned out to be total fabrication.[30] It described a 'first', the removal of an ectopic embryo from the fallopian tube, placement of the embryo in the uterus, and the ultimate delivery of a normal birth at term.

Images and responses

How does the medical profession in general respond to the images of science outlined so far? One answer is that the negative ones are commonly ignored, even though the number and diversity of these cast a significant shadow over the entire profession. There are, after all, doctors who just take comfort in the heroic side of medicine, and in their belief that they generally have congenial relationships with patients. Moreover, others do not see negative images as anything they can deal with, though they at least hope that tightening peer review and more vigorous vetting by Ethics Review Bodies will deal with issues. Others, however, often more reflective, recognise that the public needs a better understanding of the nature of medicine, how science is applied and the limits of science; maybe, too, lay people should be invited as collaborators in research.

Unfortunately, relatively little public discussion exists on such matters, and on the extent to which public education about medical science is the responsibility of the medical profession and of individual practitioners.[31] Certainly, there is much to be said to support the view that the physician's role as scientist must include being an effective expositor of medical science, to be able to explain to individual patients, and to the wider public, the many contradictions that appear in the media, the uncertainties of medical science, the nature of tests and their role in diagnosis, and more. The role of communicator (*see* Chapter 3) must be considered inseparable from this role as medical scientist.

Endnotes

1 For roles identified see Chapter 1. It is noteworthy that not all sections of the public surveyed during the EFPO project identified 'scientist', which perhaps reflected the ambivalence noted below. In, for example, Working Papers 9, 10, 14 and 16 (circulated typescripts), 'scientist' was either not identified or some characteristics associated with the term were included under lifelong learner-scholar or medical expert.

2 For a sense of how public attitudes reflect particular practices, and the interests of sociologists in such attitudes, Calnan M and Williams S (1992) Images of scientific medicine. *Sociology of Health & Illness*. **14**: 233–54.

3 *Globe and Mail*, 6 November 1997 and other newspapers. The report still reverberates through the Internet with many condemnations, for example 'Frankenstein fears after head transplant' or 'This is medical technology run completely mad and out of proportion to what's needed': www.news.bbc.co.uk/1/hi/health/1263758.stm (accessed July 2004).

4 Mistrust can be documented many times over. Patrick Bateson, vice-president of the British Royal Society, has noted, for example, that the 'public has a perception that science is out of control'. Reported in *The Scientist*, 11 June 2002: www.biomed central.com/news/20020611/4 (accessed June 2003).

5   Nowadays, Halls (or galleries) of Fame abound, often in academic institutions, though the only national Medical Hall of Fame is in Canada. Although not restricted to scientists or physician–scientists, these categories are far and away the most prominent. (*See also* Chapter 2, reference to heroes in the Golden Age of Medicine.)

6   Brieger G (1987) A portrait of surgery. Surgery in America, 1875–1889. *Surgical Clinics of North America.* **67**: 1181–216 (quote, p. 1187).

7   Altman LK (1998) *Who Goes First? The Story of Self-Experimentation in Medicine.* University of California Press, Berkeley. Criticism exists of the value of self-experimentation in that the experimenter cannot be objective.

8   From Holub M (1990) *Vanishing Lung Syndrome.* Oberlin College Press, Field Translation Series 16 (Trans. D Young and D Hábová), Oberlin, pp. 69–71.

9   Taken from Porter R (1998) *The Greatest Benefit to Mankind: a medical history of humanity.* Norton, New York, pp. 679–80.

10 Peabody FW (1930) *Doctor and Patient: papers on the relationship of the physician to men and institutions.* The Macmillan Company, New York, p. 37.

11 Lewis S (1925) *Arrowsmith.* Harcourt, Brace and Company, New York, p. 354. (Reprint Classics of Medicine Library, Gryphon Editions, New Jersey, 2001.) The same sentiment is illustrated in a recent movie, *Medicine Man* (1992). When Dr Campbell proposed giving the last of his cancer curing serum to a young boy when he was unsure whether he would be able to prepare a further batch out of his rainforest research, he was told 'you have the cure for the plague of the century [cancer] – it belongs to the human race, not to one sick kid.'

12 Lewis (1925) *Arrowsmith*, p. 392.

13 Markel H (2001) Prescribing Arrowsmith. Introduction to reprint of Lewis S (1925) *Arrowsmith*, p. 5. Among others who acknowledge having been influenced by *Arrowsmith*, see Gest H (1991) Dr Martin Arrowsmith: scientist and medical hero. *Perspectives in Biology and Medicine.* **35**: 116–24.

14 Dans PE (2000) *Doctors in the Movies: boil the water and just say aah.* Medi-Ed, Bloomington, p. 116. Dans' account also includes the views of Dr Moser, who, as 'Dr Gus Nikolais', was played by Ustinov.

15 Postcard in author's collection. The card (2000) was published by REPOhistory, a group of artists and scholars in New York during the 1990s that raised questions about the 'construction of history, to provide multiple viewpoints that encourage viewers to think critically, to explore how histories and their interpretations affect us today, and to engage with specific communities in order to facilitate their efforts to construct their own public histories.' www.repohistory.org/repo/repo_who.php3 (accessed June 2003).

16 The work of Borland is described in Schwarz L (2003) Parallel experience: how art and art theory can inform ethics in human research. *Medical Humanities Edition of the Journal of Medical Ethics.* **29** (2): 59–64.

17 The constant attacks on the behaviour of the pharmaceutical industry are among the most potent forces raising uncertainties about the morality of medicine. Any number of reflections of the concerns can be cited. For instance, in a special theme issue of the *British Medical Journal*, 2003; **326** (31 May), and Fonda D and Kivat B (2004) Curbing the drug marketeers. *Time* (Canadian edition). **164** (July 5): 26–8.

18 For the novel as a bioethics text, Davies H (2004) Can Mary Shelley's *Frankenstein* be read as an early research ethics text? *Medical Humanities Edition of the Journal of Medical Ethics.* **30** (1): 32–5.

19 The movie *The Terminator* (1984), about a cyborg, received some critical acclaim (more than its sequel, *Terminator 2: Judgment Day*) for taking science fiction seriously, for instance that the plot rests on internally driven logic. It is noteworthy that 'serious' science fiction is used in schools and universities to raise scientific concepts and ethical issues, and also to consider how science is represented in popular culture.

20 Nourse A (1974) *Bladerunner.* McKay, New York.

21 From Shoppers Drug Mart; advertisement posted in a bus shelter (St John's, Newfoundland), September 1996.

22 There are various thought-provoking discussions such as by the widely read and challenging critic, Postman N (1993) *Technopoly: the surrender of culture to technology.* Knopf, New York. Some see such works as 'technology bashers'; however, Postman, for

example, captures many concerns of other critics about the roles of technology in concluding: 'Would American medicine be better were it not so totally reliant on the technologies in practice? Here the answer is clearly, yes.'

23   Campo R (1994) *The Other Man Was Me: a voyage to the New World*. Arte Publico Press– University of Houston, Houston; also Campo's commentary quoted below: www. endeavor.med.nyu.edu/lit-med/lit-med-db/webdocs/poems/technology.medicine.rc. html (accessed July 2004).

24   Selzer R (1982) *Letters to a Young Doctor*. Simon and Schuster, New York, pp. 155–62.

25   Djerassi C (1989) *Cantor's Dilemma*. Doubleday, New York, p. 149.

26   Ibid., p. 228 from Djerassi's Afterword. Djerassi is interested in the 'trimming' of results, for instance omission in published results that, say, one rat out of seven did not survive.

27   Djerassi C (1998) *Menachem's Seed*. Penguin, New York, p. ix.

28   For notice of these and one consequence, Commentary (2004) The *Lancet*'s policy on conflicts of interest – 2004. *Lancet*. **363**: 2–3.

29   Lock S and Wells F (eds) (1993) *Fraud and Misconduct in Medical Research*. BMJ Publishing Group, London, pp. ix, 9. It is noteworthy that the volume came under the imprint of the *British Medical Journal*. Medical journalists at the time were clearly taking note of public concerns.

30   Pierce JM, Manyanda IT and Chamberlain GVP (1994) Term delivery after intrauterine relocation of an ectopic pregnancy. *British Journal of Obstetrics and Gynaecology*. **101**: 716–17. For one discussion, Lock S (1995) Lessons from the Pearce affair: handling scientific fraud. Belatedly, Britain should abandon its lax approach to scientific fraud. *British Medical Journal*. **310**: 1547–8.

31   Such questions can be sharpened by consideration of the work of historians such as Burnham JC (1987) *How Superstition Won and Science Lost: popularizing science and health in the United States*. Rutgers University Press, New Brunswick. Burnham bemoans the increasing distortion of science by the twentieth-century media, just as many others are concerned about the decline in standards of science reporting.

CHAPTER 6

Physician as health advocate: following or leading?

Introduction

'You can't look away any more' captioned a 1993 photograph of Matuschka's radical mastectomy that appeared on the cover of the *New York Times Magazine* (circulation almost two million). The photograph, taken by Matuschka herself, is mentioned here not for its contribution to the cancer wars, but as a reflection of women's involvement in a grass roots, wellness movement.[1] The latter, with an emphasis on prevention and taking control of one's health, became conspicuous during the last decades of the twentieth century as a lay movement, rather than one driven by healthcare professionals. Matuschka's own website challenges:

> Artists are messengers. The truth can be shocking and uncomfortable, but it still beats, tricks, lies and issues in disguise. The new art seeks to bring about changes in the way we practice personal politics and medicine. I created these images because I care very much about the people who have had to cope with breast cancer in their lives, in particular the women who have been subjected to irreversible, unacceptable and unnecessary methods of treatment.[2]

Matuschka is just one of countless visual artists who raise awareness of health and environmental issues through their work. Although the precise impact of this is impossible to measure, it can be seen as spotlighting, if not consolidating, issues; landscape art in Britain, for instance, is recognised as a long-standing counter-current to industrialisation.[3]

The wellness movement draws on diverse public wishes for a healthy environment that include, for example, efforts to control pollution, a search for the innate spirituality in natural places, and interest in herbs since they are natural and free from synthetic chemicals that are foreign to the body. The breadth of issues in the wellness movement prompts questions about exactly what does the public want when they expect physicians to be health advocates. Do they want physicians to embrace more than broad public health campaigns such as anti-smoking, mass vaccination and so on? Do they see physicians as overly slow in responding to public concerns?

This chapter, in offering some response to the questions, focuses particularly on concerns with the environment and health – past and present – as just one illustration of deep-seated health issues in society that call for public debate.

The environment and health

> A smell filled the Chrysler like the sharp smell of battery acid and onion fields. The smog never seemed to blow away anymore these days, as it used to even ten years ago. When the Air Pollution Control Board couldn't bring down the level of emissions they raised the limits. People kept on breathing thicker and thicker poison and fooled themselves that the air was getting cleaner. He smiled wryly. A sour taste rose out of his belly and stung his throat. A testament to old compromises.[4]

Linking the environment to health or illness was far from new when it became an increasingly conspicuous issue amid the social challenges of the 1960s; in fact, it has been part of Western medicine since its origins in ancient Greece. Over many centuries, physicians were conspicuous in advocating a healthy environment – for instance, paying attention to air, dampness, winds and cold, etc. Amid a vast amount of literature that documents this long history, 'The Art of Preserving Health', a didactic poem by poet–physician John Armstrong (1709–1779), is of particular interest. It is not only a significant historical document, but also a masterpiece of blank verse that continues to attract students. The illustrative excerpt in endnote 5 voices a long-standing, still widely held popular association between the weather and catching a cold. John Aitkin's edition of the poem is additionally noteworthy for students of medical humanities, for the editor added his own thoughts on the role of didactic poetry in health education. He believed that, in promoting the imagination, it was a good educational tool by making dull advice more pleasing.[6]

Especially relevant to our present account is that, by the end of the 1800s, many physicians were paying less attention to such long-standing environmental factors as climate, dampness, wind, etc., even while commercial/entrepreneurial pro-motion of health was becoming increasingly conspicuous. This cannot be explored here, although T Coraghessan Boyle's novel *The Road to Wellville* (1993), and the 1994 movie based on the novel, merit mention for telling a story about the activities of John Harvey Kellogg, a representative of the new commercialism; although Boyle's story is essentially entertaining satire on people's preoccupation with digestion and bowels, it is a salutary reminder to all healthcare professionals of the lengths to which many individuals go in search of health.[7]

One reason for the diminishing attention on the part of many physicians to links between the general environment and poor health was the nineteenth-century rise in the clinico-pathological approach to diagnosis, which incorporated the germ theory of disease from the 1880s onwards. The latter did much to focus attention on specific causes and effects, rather than non-specific environmental factors. Although physicians did not ignore environmental pollution, adulterated food, industrial waste and other public health hazards, such factors came to be compartmentalised as part of the increasingly specialist discipline of public health. It is not altogether surprising, then, that twentieth-century physicians have tended to give lower priority to environmental matters and preventive care compared with learning and refining the skills necessary to diagnose primary causes of, and to treat, disease.

Analogous issues surround the emergence, by around 1900, of nutrition; as an increasingly specialist discipline it also affected health advocacy in general. As new and sophisticated nutritional knowledge mushroomed, much of it from scientific laboratories, it outstripped the interests of many physicians who, until then, largely drew on the knowledge that was part of popular culture. During the twentieth century, clinical understanding of nutrition never acquired any sense of priority in medical school curricula beyond basic knowledge of biochemistry, vitamins and minerals, and special nutrition for particular diseases and for the very sick.

If interest in the relationships between the environment and health faded in the first half of the twentieth century, it did not disappear, for there were always some activists in the field.[8] However, the re-emergence of concerns about environmental health around the 1960s owed more to public pressures than to health professionals. The impetus owed much to Rachel Carson's extraordinarily influential 1962 book, *Silent Spring*. It catalysed concerns over pollution of the land and sea, which have intensified ever since through example after example of contaminated industrial sites; the infamous saga of Love Canal in New York State (residents were evacuated from their homes in 1978) is but one example.

At the end of the century, Erin Brockovitch might be said to cap ever growing public concerns.[9] Brockovitch's mission became well known when it became the subject of a movie (*Erin Brockovitch*, 2000), which won an oscar for Julie Roberts as lead role. Despite limited formal schooling, Brockovitch became a legal assistant and the key person to line up the hundreds of plaintiffs in the small California desert town of Hinckley. The huge settlement they won against the Pacific Gas and Electric Company for contaminating the town water supply has not stemmed questions as to whether the contamination actually caused ill-health – an example of the controversy and uncertainty surrounding so many cases of alleged environmental dangers in which unassailable 'scientific' proof of cause and effect is absent.

> My central nervous system is where the worst results of this interior toxic spill show themselves. Trying to wash a soup pot in the kitchen sink, I've extended the rinsing hose and pointed its nozzle down the neck of my shirt instead of into the pot, drenching and astonishing myself in an instant. I've put talcum powder instead of Crest on my toothbrush ... (Floyd Skloot)[10]

Medical humanities not only illuminates the broad sweep of environmental concerns, but also subtle effects on individuals. Author Floyd Skloot's reference to a toxic spill to describe his efforts to cope with chronic fatigue syndrome points to the pervasive impact of environmental issues on countless people.

Of particular interest and influence is Don DeLillo's award-winning novel, *White Noise*. Published in 1985, it continues – due partly to increasing environmental concerns – to arouse popular and scholarly interest.[11] One commentator has pointed out that the book reflects a quarter-century advance beyond Rachel Carson's *Silent Spring* because it takes for granted the chemical assault on health to which Carson first called attention. Yet, while a cloud of Nyodene D, 'the airborne toxic event', is the central disaster in the novel and is another warning that toxic substances are all around us, DeLillo's multi-layered story focuses on individual responses. DeLillo's challenge is to prompt readers to consider whether environmental contamination covers common, almost invisible (but potentially no less injurious) contaminants of contemporary life – station wagons, supermarkets, consumerism, drugs, expressways, and so on. Do they contribute to the white noise, the unvarying background noise in our daily lives?[12] Such noise becomes accepted and remains unobtrusive to many, but for others it contributes to 'let's get away from it all' feelings, the need of retreats and spas, and even to interest in 'natural' rather than 'artificial' foods and medicines.

DeLillo's novel raises a number of specific issues. For instance, while Babette Gladney regularly runs up and down the stairs of a football stadium to keep her weight down, it is the marketing of disease, of treatments, that envelops her. Babette is haunted by a new disease, 'fear of death', which led her on an endless search for information and help, even to studying the occult. Unknown to her husband, Jack Gladney, or to her physician, she tried an experimental psychoactive drug, Dylar, in consequence of responding to an 'ad' in the *National Examiner* – 'volunteers wanted for secret research'. It turned out that a trial was felt to be too risky, but by a private 'arrangement' with the project manager – regular assignations with him in a grubby motel room – Babette obtained a regular supply as a 'last resort'. She hoped that her condition, with a key symptom of memory loss, would be fixed by the drug.[13] The latter, a creation of the pharmaceutical industry, was described as a 'superbly engineered' wonder of pharmaceutical technology:

> It's a drug delivery system. It doesn't dissolve right away or release its ingredients right away. The medication in Dylar is encased in a polymer membrane. Water from your gastrointestinal tract seeps through the membrane at a carefully controlled rate [to dissolve] the medication encased in the membrane. Slowly, gradually, precisely. The medicine then passes out of the polymer tablet through a single small hole [which is] laser-drilled. It's not only tiny but stunningly precise in its dimensions.'[14]

Such pharmaceutical 'wonders', backed by massive pharmaceutical advertising that is a reality in the non-fictional world, are but one contribution to the 'white noise' of commercialism. A particular issue, increasingly commented on since the 1990s, is that pharmaceutical companies continually look for new diseases or new 'conditions' in order to extend the market for their drugs – a topic that has aroused diverse commentaries from the irreverent movie *Brain Candy* (1996) to first-class media reporting.[15] The intimate links between commercialism, consumerism and healthcare can be very much part of life today and very much part of DeLillo's white noise.

The domestic environment

Someone once told me that we never remember pain. Once it's gone it's gone. A nurse. She told me just before the doctor put my arm back in its socket. She was being nice. She's seen me before.

– fell down the stairs again, I told her. – Sorry.

No questions asked. What about the burn on my hand? The missing hair? The teeth? I waited to be asked. Ask me. Ask me. I'd tell her. I'd tell them everything. Look at the burn. Ask me about it. Ask.[16]

Roddy Doyle's novel, *The Woman Who Walked Into Doors*, centres on spousal abuse. The 'patient' goes on with her story of the hospital visit by noting that the doctor never 'looked at me.' He had already decided that it was a problem with alcohol. 'He studied parts of me, but he never saw all of me.'

A conspicuous aspect of healthcare in the second half of the twentieth century has been the expansion of its boundaries into areas not always considered 'medical'. Social trends behind this often invoke the advocacy of the World Health Organization, namely that maximum health is dependent on attention to psychological and social conditions as much as to the physical aspects of an illness. Amidst this, 'domestic' issues – ranging from spousal and child abuse (physical and mental) to sick-building syndrome – have become very much part of environmental issues in general.

Although professional writings have done much to raise awareness of spousal and child abuse, storytellers, with the practised eye of the observer, can voice lessons more telling than found in medical textbooks. Another quote from Roddy Doyle's novel reminds us that the battered wife has many feelings common to other victims: 'For seventeen years. There wasn't one minute, when I wasn't afraid, when I wasn't waiting. Waiting for him to go, waiting for him to come, waiting for the fist, waiting for the smile. I was brainwashed, a zombie for hours, afraid to think, afraid to stop, completely alone.'[17]

One consequence of concerns with domestic violence is that physicians and other healthcare professionals now have legislated responsibilities to report cases to public authorities. This can often open up many moral and clinical challenges in differentiating assault from accidents, tendencies to stereotype people, and so on. One is again reminded of the dilemmas unearthed in the 'Playing God' story by Michael LaCombe (*see* Chapter 2).

Physician responsibilities: following or leading?

Given the challenges posed by the environment and by other public health issues, we return to a query that opened this chapter about physicians' responsibilities. Has medicine in recent times been overly slow in responding to public concerns? Have physicians been content to leave the advocacy in the hands of lay individuals such as Carson, Brockovitch, DeLillo, Matuschka and countless other activists? It is, after all, fairly clear that the public would welcome authoritative, independent advice from its experts in healthcare, given the availability of so much commercially driven contradictory advice.

It is unfortunate that, as noted, environmental/public health issues in the hands of physicians have tended to take second place to diagnosis and treatment of individuals, even if they stayed on the radar screen so to speak. It is, too, nowadays easy for physicians to feel overwhelmed by the expanding medical system. Thus it has been said:

> There I am standing by the shore of a swiftly flowing river and I hear the cry of a drowning man. So I jump into the river, put my arms around him, pull him to shore and apply artificial respiration. Just when he

begins to breathe, there is another cry for help. So I jump into the river, reach him, pull him to shore, apply artificial respiration, and then just as he begins to breathe, another cry for help. So back in the river again, reaching, pulling, applying, breathing and then another yell. Again and again, without end, goes the sequence. You know, I am so busy jumping in, pulling them to shore, applying artificial respiration, that I have no time to see who is upstream pushing them all in.[18]

As an aside, it is unfortunately also true that, given the complexity of research protocols nowadays, few physicians have the ready opportunity that contributed to the fame of, for example, John Snow (1813–1858). His 1854 study of cholera deaths led him to one of the most celebrated events in the history of public health. On observing that most victims had used the local Broad Street pump in the Soho district of London, he concluded that, rather than being spread by a poison in the air, cholera was transmitted by the local water supply. By persuading the parish authorities to remove the pump handle, his ideas were confirmed by a dramatic drop in the incidence of cases.

One particular issue nowadays is ethical dilemmas over potential clashes of interests that can inhibit the commitment of some physicians to whistle blowing on, say, an environmental issue. A physician who draws attention to an industrial hazard may well put workers (perhaps the doctor's own patients) out of work – a clash of interests that can extend to problems between industry and researchers.[19]

Yet given the central place of physicians and other healthcare workers in healthcare systems, it can be viewed as ostrich-like for physicians to step back from general health issues. A noteworthy essay, 'Lead, follow or get out of the way: What is the physician's role in a changing society?' (1996) by medical student Matthew Rose, suggested that the medical profession has two options in responding to social issues that affect health. It can either recognise the demands of modern society and plan for more responsive and responsible healthcare, or it can try to protect its own interests and turf and adapt to changes only when it has no other choice.[20]

Rose raises the particular question: to what extent does the medical profession commit to healthcare at the societal level? After all, questions have been raised in the past and continue about the slow responsiveness (some say conservatism) of medicine to healthcare reform. Although many individual physicians have been proactive, the medical profession as a whole is commonly viewed as always being slow in taking a leadership role.[21] A central issue is the long-standing ethic that the physician's responsibility is to his or her individual patients, a responsibility underpinned by confidentiality. One physician's response to Rose's article stated: 'I hope that *my* physician is an old reactionary and will consider my interests first [rather than society's] when giving me important advice.'[22]

The question, then, is how proactive should physicians be, even with, for example, such national/local health programmes as anti-smoking and anti-obesity? Should such programmes be pursued more vigorously than placing posters on waiting-room walls or mild admonishments to patients? And must they be role models? Advice, obviously, has a hollow ring when the physician is overweight or a smoker. Moreover, good role models may worry about being particularly proactive with health programmes that can be perceived as 'blaming' patients for their ill-health; some physicians may agree with the view that, as blaming became increasingly noticeable in the last years of the twentieth century, it has become one of the 'most disturbing aspects of the contemporary health promotion movement.'[23] Health education programmes directed to medical conditions linked to obesity, smoking and alcohol have not escaped the charge of being intolerant, self-righteous and punitive.[24]

The contentious issue of blaming serves as a reminder that formal medical education provides little instruction in understanding the diversity of lay beliefs and of lifestyles where risk behaviour is, in many ways, the norm. Perhaps no textbook matches many essays and novels in exploring the complexity of human relationships. As an example, Hanif Kureshi's insights in *The Black Album* certainly offer a sense that, for some people, taking drugs and risks is a natural part of certain lifestyles.[25]

In closing this chapter, it must be added that despite what many see as a modest response to social concerns on the part of the medical profession as a whole, there has always been a vigorous core of physicians who view environmental matters and health promotion seriously and are active in its promotion. Some in following, sometimes leading, public voices belong to organisations that challenge all physicians, indeed underscore questions about what social values physicians hold. In 1985 the Nobel Peace Prize was awarded to the International Physicians for the Prevention of Nuclear War. In part this was for creating an awareness of the catastrophic consequences of atomic warfare. As one of the acceptance speeches stated: 'We physicians who shepherd human life from birth to death have a moral imperative to resist with all our being the drift toward the brink. The threatened inhabitants on this fragile planet must speak out for those yet unborn [,] for prosperity has no lobby with politicians.'[26] In the early 1990s, the affiliated Physicians for Social Responsibility expanded activism in health issues. Its 1993 goal-setting work *Critical Condition: Human Health and the Environment* remains as a *magna carta*.[27] The authors argue that all physicians (especially primary care physicians) need to understand the relationship of environment to health. They should be able to detect and diagnose environmentally related disease, know how to obtain information about environmental hazards, advise patients on intervention strategies to reduce exposure to environmental hazards, and be able to refer patients to specialists in environmental and occupational medicine. It is noteworthy that the *British Medical Journal* did underscore climate and health issues as a response to the 2004 Hollywood movie *The Day After Tomorrow*, which presents the worst-case scenario (a condensed time period) of weather-related disasters on New York City resulting from climate change.[28]

As a last summary remark in this chapter, health advocacy, perhaps more so than other roles discussed in this book, challenges physicians to enlarge the boundaries of their already complex practices and responsibilities. Apart from such matters as environmental issues and spouse battering (already noted), a whole range of lifestyle considerations, from medications to cosmetic surgery, challenge physicians to consider their own values with respect to patients and medical care and the pressures on their own lifestyles; at the very least to consider whether social activism should be part of professional values.

Endnotes

1   The photograph appeared on 15 August 1993. See also the Matuschka website: www. songster.net/projects/matuschka/matuschka_invasive.html (accessed July 2004. For context in connection with the cancer wars, Lerner BH (2001) *The Breast Cancer Wars: hope, fear, and the pursuit of a cure in twentieth-century America.* Oxford University Press, Oxford.

2   www.songster.net/projects/matuschka/matuschka_invasive.html (accessed November 2002).

3   For a discussion on issues today, Peat FD 'Art and the Environment in Britain': www. fdavidpeat.com/bibliography/essays/artbrit.htm (accessed June 2004). Some historical perspectives are also made clear in the 2004 exhibition 'Turner, Whistler, Monet'. See catalogue, Lochnan K (ed) (2004) *Turner, Whistler, Monet: Impressionist visions.* Tate Publishing, London.

4   Quote from Campbell R (1986) *In La-La Land We Trust.* The Mysterious Press, New York, p. 120. Taken from 'Literature/Attitudes to Los Angeles Air Pollution': www.uea.ac.uk/~e490/e3c62/quote.htm (accessed July 2004).

5   But may no fogs, from lake or fenny plain,
    Involve my hill! And wheresoe'er you build;
    Whether on sun-burnt Epsom, or the plains
    Wash'd by the silent Lee; in Chelsea low,
    Or high Blackheath with wintry winds assail'd;
    Dry be your house: but airy more than warm.
    Else every breath of ruder wind will strike
    Your tender body thro' with rapid pains;
    Fierce coughs will teize you, hoarseness bind your voice,
    Or moist Gravedo load your aching brows.
    These to defy, and all the fates that dwell
    In cloister'd air, tainted with steaming life,
    Let lofty ceilings grace your ample rooms;
    And still at azure noontide may your dome
    At every window drink the liquid sky.

    Armstrong J (1744) *The Art of Preserving Health: a poem.* A Millar, London, pp. 19–20. (Reprint Arno Press, New York, 1979.)

6   Armstrong J (1796) *The Art of Preserving Health* (ed J Aitkin). Cadell and Davies, London. Editor's introduction.

7   Boyle TG (1993) *The Road to Wellville.* Viking, New York.

8   For some account of interest, Sargent II F (1982) *Hippocratic Heritage: a history of ideas about weather and human health.* Pergamon, New York.

9   Noteworthy, too, is the best-selling non-fiction, Harr J (1996) *A Civil Action.* Random House, New York, that relates a true story of water pollution in Woburn, Massachussetts, and a high incidence of childhood leukaemia. The movie, based on the book and with the same title, appeared in 1998.

10 Skloot F (1996) *The Night-Side: chronic fatigue syndrome and the illness experience.* Story Line Press, Brownsville, p. 4. Skloot writes about his experiences with chronic fatigue syndrome.

11 Osteen M (ed) (1998) *Don DeLillo White Noise.* Penguin Books, New York. (Full text of novel and various commentaries.) Interest remains high at the level of university education.

12 Morris DB (1996) Environment: the white noise of health. *Literature and Medicine.* **15**: 1–15.

13 Osteen M (ed) (1998) *Don DeLillo White Noise,* pp. 196 and 202.

14 Ibid., pp. 187–8.

15 This has been raised a number of times, e.g. Payer L (1992) *Disease Mongers: how doctors, drug companies, and insurers are making you feel sick.* Wiley, New York. In 2003, a book with a similar theme became a best seller in Germany, see review by A Tufts on Blech J (2003) Die Krankheitserfinder: Wie Wir zu Patienten Gemacht Werden. *British Medical Journal.* **327**: 1173.

16 Doyle R (1997) *The Woman Who Walked Into Doors*. Minerva, London, p. 164.

17 Ibid., p. 176.

18 Zola IK (1970) Helping – does it matter: the problems and prospects of mutual aid groups. Address to the United States Ostomy Association, 1970. In: Alonzo AA (1993) Health behavior: issues, contradictions and dilemmas. *Social Science and Medicine*. **37**: 1019–34.

19 Clashes between researchers and the industries that finance research have become an increasing issue. One illustrative case involved an occupational health physician at Brown University, David Kern. As part of a consulting agreement, he evaluated a number of workers from a local nylon flocking plant. During the study he diagnosed several workers with interstitial lung disease. He learned that researchers in Canada had previously found a similarly high incidence of interstitial lung disease in another plant utilising the same processes and owned by the same company. Kern actively undertook to fulfil his obligations to report, informing the company and the National Institute for Occupational Safety and Health of his findings. In addition, he prepared a paper describing his investigation and the results to date to be delivered at an upcoming conference. This is consistent with item 15 of the International Commission on Occupational Health Code of Ethics which states that occupational health professionals must report objectively to the scientific community on new or suspected occupational hazards and relevant preventive methods. In fact, the University did not support Kern, who left academia as a disillusioned whistle-blower. (Shuchman M (2000) Consequences of blowing the whistle in medical research. *Annals of Internal Medicine*. **132**: 1013–15.)

20 Rose M (1996) Lead, follow or get out of the way: what is the physician's role in a changing society? *Canadian Medical Association Journal*. **155**: 209–11.

21 For discussion on Canada, not irrelevant to elsewhere, Stevenson HM and Williams AP (1988) Physicians and medicare: professional ideology and Canadian health-care policy. In: Bolaria BS and Dickinson HD (eds) *Sociology of Healthcare in Canada*. Harcourt Brace Jovanovich, Toronto, pp. 92–102.

22 Duic AD (1996) Whose interest? Patient's, physician's or society's? *Canadian Medical Association Journal*. **155**: 1236. For other letters, ibid., pp. 1235–6.

23 Becker MH (1986) The tyranny of health promotion. *Public Health Reviews*. **14**: 15–25. In: Woods S, Ritzel DO and Drolet JC (1996) Blaming the victim: selected college students' health and illness causation beliefs. *Journal of Health Education*. **27**: 228–34.

24 Kilwein JH (1989) No pain, no gain: a puritan legacy. *Health Education Quarterly*. **16**: 9–12. In: Alonzo AA (1993) Health behavior: issues, contradictions and dilemmas. *Social Science and Medicine*. **37**: 1019–34.

25 Kureshi H (1995) *The Black Album*. Scribner, New York. It is appropriate to add that attitudes to AIDS offer many lessons about how lay beliefs and urban legends shape attitudes and behaviours. Cf., for example, Goldstein DE (ed) (1991) *Talking Aids: interdisciplinary perspectives on acquired inmmune deficiency syndrome*. Iser Research and Policy Papers, St John's, Newfoundland.

26 Quoted from Dr Bernard Lown's acceptance speech: www.ippnw.org/Lown.html (accessed July 2004).

27 Chivian E, McCally M, Hu H and Haines A (eds) (1993) *Critical Condition: human health and the environment*. MIT Press, Cambridge, MA.

28 For introduction and references to other relevant pages in the issue, Smith R (2004) Cataclysm and departure. *British Medical Journal*. **328**: 1268.

CHAPTER 7

A team member

Teams and hierarchies

> My wife was marvellous. She was what I call my memory. She knew the
> community better than I did. She knew who was related to who and
> she could tie in anything for me. She knew whose wake I should go to,
> she knew all kinds of things that directed me in this way. It was very
> much a team thing. Again, my family, my children would come with me
> on housecalls, on rounds. And they would come out of the car and play
> with the kids while I went in and did business and came out again, and
> I would often leave them there while I went on to the other houses
> because they were enjoying it; they were also part of this same com-
> munity and how to communicate the value of that to students I find very
> difficult. It's even difficult to show them yourself when living it. (Dr John
> Ross, General Practitioner, 1995)[1]

Husband–wife (frequently doctor–nurse) or family 'teams', very much part of the
lore and history of general practice, have all but disappeared from contemporary
medicine. This is a consequence of diverse social changes that range from doctors
now marrying doctors (rather than nurses) to the emergence of the 'new' patient,
and of patients' rights. Relevant, too, are changes in patterns of care that relate not
only to developments in medicine, but also, by the 1970s or so, to social changes,
such as improved transport in far-flung rural areas. As one Canadian general
practitioner noted in 1989: 'I think the greatest change in medicine on these islands
[in rural Newfoundland] is that no longer do we feel self-sufficient, that we should
do everything the patient needs ... We refer our patients to other specialists, to
tertiary centres where the high-intensity medical care is given.'[2]

•

In looking at the current interest in team care and public demands that physicians
be part of a team, this chapter is short, for the voices of the humanities have offered
relatively little direct comment. This is despite intense public interest reflected, at
least in part, on the World Wide Web – a Google search for healthcare teams in June
2004 elicited over 2 million hits.

It is noteworthy that the early 1990s survey on public expectations of physicians
identified not the role of 'team player', but of 'manager/gatekeeper'. This was in
keeping with less attention, compared with nowadays, given to the notion of
integrated team care. Concerns were primarily about poor communication between
healthcare professionals, all of whom might be involved in the care of a patient.
Further, frustrations existed that physicians, who controlled or filtered access to

other healthcare practitioners, were not always adequately informed or even respectful of other services available to patients. Views were expressed that physicians were territorial and protective of their 'expert' status, even reluctant to refer patients to other physicians for a second opinion.[3] Yet clearly such concerns helped to open doors to concepts of team care. Further, during the 1990s, gatekeeping was increasingly scrutinised in the context of, for instance, the patients' rights movement, demands for patients to have a greater say in healthcare, and calls from the nursing profession for team care.

Some of the interest in team care also stems from public demands for 'integrated care'. Although this term is used in various contexts, including integrated patient services from conventional practitioners, it has been popularised through efforts of individuals to integrate complementary and alternative medicine with conventional medicine. The needs of certain patients for such integration are implicit in, for example, Floyd Skloot's *The Night-Side*, a collection of essays describing his experiences with disabling chronic fatigue syndrome.[4] Although Skloot makes clear that coping is personal, his concerns over clinical trials and his uncertain attitudes toward complementary/alternative practices voice a need for help with the diversity of healthcare options, in other words, a call for team care. Ruminating on his 'trial' of the ayurvedic-based regimen of Panchakarma, he perceptively noted a telling dilemma for many patients: 'I was a classic case of a person whose mind and body are working at cross purposes in the healing process. Here were these people trying to unleash my body's own healing powers and I was hindering them by using symptom warfare.'[5]

Other voices, increasingly heard by the early 2000s, called for spiritual care to be incorporated into conventional medicine as part of integrated team care. This includes, for example, not only asking that physicians take a patient's spiritual history, especially in the context of healing (*see* Chapter 4), but also that specially trained pastoral care professionals (mostly clergy with additional training in healthcare situations) be a part of clinical team care. Many patients now find that the latter's involvement in team care is variable, even though those specially trained in pastoral care within healthcare settings can serve the needs of countless patients, including those who do not identify themselves with any particular faith group.[6] Novelists have explored issues of spirituality and health from various directions. Ron Querry's *Bad Medicine* (1998) is one of many voices spotlighting the relationships of culture and health for native people in North America. Querry calls for integration of care beyond the immediate needs of individuals. Based on a hantavirus outbreak among native people in the southwestern United States, *Bad Medicine* leaves readers in no doubt that conventional and traditional medicine must collaborate to take care not only of individual patients, but also of the environment as an important health determinant.[7]

Should patients be members of the team?

An implicit, if not explicit question, in many commentaries on healthcare is whether the patient should be a member of the team. One of LaCombe's masterful stories, 'The Bag Lady', a fable about lay healing, tells of the impact of a mysterious patient on all the members of a medical team.[8] From the medical student to the attending physician, the bag lady helped them all to reflect on themselves, on their own personal lives. 'The hospital had never seen a more peculiar patient.' She was an enigma as reflected in various notes written in her chart by the legions of doctors who, over time, had examined her: 'this young Hispanic from the west coast enters with a chief complaint of ... This is the first admission for this Eastern European teacher of thirty-seven ... This fifty-four-year-old white New Englander complains of ...' Her illness was equally ill-defined. Dressed like a sack of dirty laundry, she had all the makings of being a 'difficult patient', but 'everyone at the hospital found her immensely compelling without being able to state precisely why.'

As the doctors and students surrounded her bed in the formality of a teaching hospital, 'the woman nodded a silent greeting to her new physicians, fixing each in turn with her steady look.' The senior physician, in considering his new patient, escaped from her gaze by tearing his eyes away 'to scan the notes in her medical record.' Each member of the team found a strange connection with the woman in the bed. Each felt that it was he or she being scrutinised, dissected, laid bare. And such was her aura that each one saw her in a different way.

LaCombe made it clear that each member of the team found particular connections depending on their personal needs. For instance, Marianne Rehnicke, the medical student, experienced a 'surge of emotion – a wave of affection that rose from a place buried as deep within her as her earliest memories. This was someone, she thought, in whom she could confide. She became filled with unaccustomed trust. Here was the friend she had been looking for.' No one who entered the bag lady's room left untouched. Just how her calming presence touched the psyche of each of them depended on their own desires and defences. But as the story suggests, they were forced to ponder how they felt. Some who visited – Nurse Costigan, for one – were so far distanced from themselves that they could only think of the haunting apprehension of disorder. Others, like Marianne, were personally profoundly affected

Although the bag lady was in no way a member of the team, her presence fulfilled one role of a team player – helping other members to reflect on themselves and their own roles. The story theme contrasts sharply with a painting by Robert Pope, completed while he was a cancer patient. It depicts looking through a door into a patient's room from the corridor where three white-coated physicians, standing far away from the patient, just outside the door, consulted with each other, presumably about the patient.[9] The question arises, to what extent does the bag lady and Pope's painting challenge views expressed in a recent textbook on team care: '[while a] patient's needs are central to the team's focus, and a patient or designee must be an active participant in the team's work ... it is disingenuous to consider the patient a member of an interdisciplinary health team that needs to work on its tasks and processes for healthcare delivery'?[10] Many will suggest that this smacks of old paternalism.

Barriers to team care

Physician Robert Burns' one-act play, *A Simple Procedure*, takes place in a patient's room in a suburban teaching hospital.[11] It describes a conversation between Sarah Williams, aged 72 and neatly dressed in a blue gown and matching robe, and Ken Porter, MD, 38 years of age who wears a wrinkled white coat. Dr Porter knocks on Sarah's door, and enters without waiting for a reply. After a brief introduction in which 'Ms' Williams is corrected to 'Mrs' Williams, Porter tells her that Dr Janson 'asked me to see you.' Sarah's retort was: 'Well she's already done that. Not to mention every medical student who's walked through those doors, as well as residents.' Dr Porter is just able to edge in the comment that he's neither student nor resident, before Sarah continues: 'You know, I may just start charging them to examine me. What would be a fair price?'

In elaborating on this, Sarah says, 'Let's say a quarter to feel my ... This is my liver over here, isn't it? ... And for my heart, it would be 50 cents. So they could listen to the murmur. That's what it's called, isn't it?' In exasperation, Porter says, 'I'm only interested in your liver.' The banter goes on with the physician trying to get across that he's a specialist. 'I'm a gastro ... I specialize in the gastrointestinal tract. The esophagus, stomach. Bowels and the liver. I mostly focus on the liver.' Sarah's inevitable response is 'Just the liver? What about the rest of the body? ... Don't you care about the rest of me?'

If the voices of the humanities, except for some autopathographies, have not been explicit in calling for team care, they have spotlighted, sometimes indirectly, many of the barriers to it. One is the entrenched role of hierarchies, which is often noted as a contentious issue between nurses and physicians, as well as the medical profession itself, especially between specialists and generalists. Specialist care has always provoked differing attitudes among patients – sometimes ambivalent, sometimes bemused, as well captured in Robert Burns' play. Not surprisingly, one response from many people to such scenarios, in which the physician is perceived to be uninterested in the 'rest of the body' or indeed the person, is to call for professionals to consciously *work together*. Often this implies overcoming hierarchies in the healthcare professions. As one senior healthcare administrator said in 1995 with regard to the Canadian scene, but equally relevant to healthcare in the US and Britain, 'hierarchies are good organizational structures in times of stability, but not in the current unstable environments of healthcare change. The issue is how to break down a hierarchy without destroying the whole thing.'[12]

Hierarchical barriers within the medical profession extend beyond uneasy specialist/generalist relations in many ways. One is the tendency of the medical profession to push into the professional desert those who do not conform to the accepted precepts and standards of the medical profession. The history of medicine is full of physicians pushed into the role of virtual 'outsiders'. One notable example is the Canadian Norman Bethune, whose heroic status in now assured in the public mind. For instance, the 1996 movie, *Dr Bethune,* reveals to the public a surgeon whose leanings towards social justice led to difficult relations with the medical establishment in Montreal. However, his activism, his pioneering of war-time blood transfusion in Spain, and his service in China, ultimately made him into a Canadian medical hero.[13] If the profession is less rigid nowadays in deciding who 'belongs', local politics may find an individual who is 'different' pushed away from the centre of the profession as Robertson Davies makes clear in his already mentioned novel, *The Cunning Man.*

Given mindsets of hierarchies, it is not surprising that, despite many positive responses toward team care from healthcare professionals, the early 2000s witnessed physicians who regarded concepts of multidisciplinary team care as a challenge to medical professionalism, at least if they were not the leader. Indeed, many issues are raised that usually receive relatively little publicity since publications describing team care generally report positive rather than negative experiences.

Anecdotal evidence certainly suggests that professional/ethical problems commonly arise, even in specialties where team care has become fairly widely established as in psychiatry, oncology and palliative care.[14] Problem areas cover not only who should be a leader of a team, but also the legal responsibilities of a leader, and the diverse moral values held among members of the team. The latter can be an issue when, for instance, a patient's competency is questioned, when relatives disagree over management of the patient, or when inappropriate dosages of sedatives are prescribed, perhaps with fears for a patient's life.

Issues surrounding team care have been compared with sports, especially the need for coaches, captains and referees. Some have contrasted healthcare teams with jazz groups where each member plays off the other, albeit guided by commonly understood principles. However, jazz groups only function with a small number of players; larger groups of musicians need conductors. Such analogies have prompted questions about rotating leaderships of a healthcare team – questions most likely to be raised by non-physician members of a team. Arguments exist to support both physician and rotating leadership. For instance, although in 1983 philosopher William May recognised that the physician's authority is precarious, he made clear that both physician authority and responsibility are much greater than that of the other members of a team. In contrast, another philosopher advocates a kind of rotating captaincy for the team, at least when complex medical and social problems exist, a captaincy that is not automatically ascribed according to rank or title, but is determined by the stage which the process of healing has reached.[15]

In closing these brief comments on team care, it has to be said that expectations of the physician's role or roles as team player are not sharply defined by the public, or indeed by the health professions, even as trends exist to develop interdisciplinary teaching for medical, nursing and pharmacy students. Patients vary in their expectations, often depending on their background and situation. However, all voices want quality care and the avoidance of disconcerting numbers of medical errors, many due to miscommunication between healthcare professionals, an issue that the medical profession now acknowledges publicly as a major problem. Many voices, in suggesting that team care can deal with this and other concerns, call on the medical profession for leadership.

Endnotes

1 Crellin JK and Curran C (1996) *Contemporary Issues – Health Care in Contemporary Canadian Society: changing direction [Philosophy 2807 by Distance Education].* Memorial University of Newfoundland School of Continuing Education, p. 3–55.
2 Comments from Newfoundland, but relevant to many other rural areas: Sheldon J (1998) Afterwords. In: Saunders GL *Doctor, When You're Sick You're Not Well: forty years of outpatient humour from Twillingate Hospital, Newfoundland.* Breakwater, St John's, p. 72.
3 For example, specifically noted in EFPO Working Paper #9, 1992, p. 12.
4 Skloot F (1996) *The Night-Side: chronic fatigue syndrome and the illness experience.* Story Line Press, Brownsville. This is not the place to expound on issues surrounding responsibilities of physicians to integrate complementary/alternative medicine into their practice, but see White A (2003) 'Is integrated medicine respectable?' *Complementary Therapies in Medicine.* **11**: 140–1.
5 Skloot (1996) *The Night-Side*, p. 129.

6   I am grateful to Rev. Peter Barnes and Rev. Bill Bartlett for perspectives on pastoral care in hospitals, its problems and potential.

7   Querry R (1998) *Bad Medicine*. Bantam Books, New York. Points made by C Belling in review in Literature, Arts and Medicine Database: www.endeavor.med.nyu.edu/lit-med/lit-med-db/webdocs/webdescrips/querry11879-des-.html (accessed June 2004).

8   LaCombe MA (1991) The bag lady. *American Journal of Medicine*. **90**: 622–7.

9   Pope R (1991) *Illness and Healing: images of cancer*. Lancelot Press, Hantsport, p. 112.

10   Drinka TJK and Clark PG (2000) *Health Care Teamwork: interdisciplinary practice and teaching*. Aubern House, Westport, p. xvii.

11   Burns R (2000) *A simple procedure: a play in one act*. In: LaCombe MA (ed) *On Being a Doctor 2: voices of physicians and patients*. American College of Physicians, Philadelphia, pp. 192–200. Also *Annals of Internal Medicine*, 1999, **130**: 158–60.

12   Quote from Sister Elizabeth Davis, Chief Executive Officer of the St John's Health Care Corporation. In Crellin and Curran *Contemporary Issues* (1996), p. 1–7.

13   While Bethune's heroic stature is now assured, a critical biography has not yet appeared. For introduction, see website of Canadian Hall of Medical Fame: www.cdnmedhall.org/laureates/?laur_id=37 (accessed July 2004).

14   Although the titles of a growing number of textbooks – e.g., *Caring for Children with Cerebral Palsy: a team-based approach* and *Ethical Patient Care: a casebook for geriatric health care teams* – suggest the team movement is well underway, various issues exist. See, for example, Randall F and Downie RS (1996) *Palliative Care Ethics: a good companion*. Oxford University Press, Oxford.

15   May WF (1983) *The Physician's Covenant: Images of the healer in medical ethics*. Westminster Press, Philadelphia, and Walker M (1997) Geographies of responsibility. *Hastings Center Report*. **27** (1): 38–44.

CHAPTER 8

Being a person

> I think that the doctor can keep his technical posture and still move into the human arena ... I see no reason why he has to stop being a doctor and become an amateur human being. Yet many doctors systematically avoid contact. (Anatole Broyard)[1]

At first sight designating one of the roles of a physician as being a 'person' – maybe best expressed as a *human* being – is perhaps a surprise. However, the role emerged, in large part, from medical students' input into the early 1990s survey (cf. Chapter 1). For various reasons, many students and young physicians were reacting to the adage, 'Medicine is a jealous mistress.'[2] Lifestyles were changing for everyone in society. Physicians were saying that they had 'rights' as persons at a time when much attention centred on the profession's high rates of alcoholism, drug addiction, burn-out and divorce (*see* Chapter 2). It is not surprising that the late 1970s saw the establishment of the Center for Professional Well-Being in the US, which remains in the vanguard of programmes for stress and burn-out for healthcare professionals.[3] Since the '70s, as already illustrated in this volume, more and more demands are being placed on medicine and on physicians so that it is not surprising that the phrase, 'the doctor is now our secular priest', is commonplace.

It has also to be appreciated that patients, too, want their doctor to be a person, at least a human being, as did Anatole Broyard (opening quote to this chapter). Moreover, patients worry about their safety whenever their physicians work excessively long hours, an issue raised in Chapter 2 with respect to stress. Reminders about this have been voiced widely for a long time. A 'bone-tired' physician appeared in a 1972 novel after 'eight hours at the operating room, two in the clinic, grand rounds, teaching rounds, and only a chocolate bar for lunch.' He was 'drained, and now that he longed to leave for the farm, this call [from the ward] had come.'[4] And, in the movie *Killer on Board* (1977), a doctor apologises for his poor 'people skills'. 'You lose contact with people in hospital. You don't know who they are.' Around the same time, physician Robin Cook, in one of the early (1972) exposés of medical school/intern life, reported that 'internship as it exists today *is* an adverse environment. (The lack of sleep alone is sufficient to explain a host of aberrant behavior patterns.)'[5] And in the British physician Jonathan Gash's medical mystery, *Prey Dancing* (1998), a central character, Dr Clare Burtonall, observed that 'books should be written about doctors' internal clocks ... The problem wasn't getting along with patients, staff, finding instruments for surgical ward procedures, knowing where the pharmacy was. The age-old problem was one's internal biorhythms. Like what to do at five-thirty in the morning in a ghostly hospital.'[6]

This chapter looks first at one broad issue, physician detachment – the mindset that a physician should not get emotionally involved with patients. This is often a concern to patients, though the voices we notice are those of physicians echoing those concerns. Next we comment on long-standing advice to physicians about reflecting on oneself as a person. This is followed by an appendix that prompts further reflection on medicine and physicians.

Clinical detachment

'What's that?' I asked my medical resident just before morning rounds began.

'It's a muffin,' she said. 'Mrs Tyler on Farnsworth Five likes muffins, especially blueberry. This one came on her tray this morning. It's so hard, I'm afraid it might crush her jaw.'

I picked it up. It did seem like a cross between a hockey puck and a golf ball. I thought little else about it and we started rounds.

A few days later we went out to breakfast to say goodbye to our medical students who were rotating off service. I still can't remember what inspired me to say, 'Let's buy a blueberry muffin for Mrs Tyler. We can drop it off on the way back to the conference room.'

We bought the muffin and stopped by her room to give it to her. Mrs Tyler was 83 years old, paraplegic from spinal stenosis, bed-bound, and suffering from a deep decubitus ulcer. Her oral intake was lousy, and we were considering a feeding tube. She was a pleasant woman, alert and quite sharp mentally. However, given her condition, she usually appeared depressed. She brightened when we presented her with the muffin. I also noticed that she was reading a Dick Francis novel.

'Do you like mystery novels?' I asked.

'All of them!' she exclaimed. As we retreated to our conference room, the housestaff informed me that she read a book every two days and was rapidly finishing the hospital's entire stash of mysteries.

So opens a short story, 'Blueberry Muffins and Mystery Novels', by physician Mark Linzer.[7] The story goes on to describe how the physician regularly took blueberry muffins and mystery novels to Mrs Tyler. When after three weeks it was suggested that she be put on a Do Not Resuscitate order, the physician was 'stopped' in his tracks:

First I nodded yes. Then I said, 'Wait a minute.' Tears welled up in my eyes. My voice caught. I tried to speak.

'I need to sort this out. I can't figure out what I'm feeling. Maybe we should talk to her' ...

I had crossed the line. My residents knew. I related to her in a more personal manner, without the 'detached concern' that is supposed to define our relationships with patients ... I also recognized that something else had occurred that day on rounds. By sharing my feelings with my team of students and housestaff, I had begun to legitimize a 'feeling process'.

Linzer is clearly challenging medical thinking about clinical detachment – avoiding involvement with a patient so as to avoid undue emotional stress that might contribute to burn-out. In so doing he is questioning the view that detachment is necessary to preserve professional judgement and behaviour; moreover, that it protects patients from potential clinical bias.[8] In contrast to physicians who feel that detachment is a necessary part of practice – even though it may undermine one's ability to be empathetic – Linzer recognized that he had to acknowledge his feelings and their relevance to patient care. In sharing with students and housestaff his legitimising of a 'feeling process', he concluded that it was right to show that the attending physician is not 'divorced from his humanity'.

Innumerable other physicians have drawn attention to the dilemma of detachment in stories and essays. Richard Selzer, for instance, in 'An Absence of Windows', questioned the wisdom of revealing emotion as he commenced exploratory surgery on the mailman in his hospital:

> 'Go to sleep, Pete,' I say into his ear [as he was being anaesthetised] so close it is almost a kiss. 'When you wake up, it will be all behind you.'
> I should not have spoken his name aloud! No good will come of it. The syllable has peeled from me something, a skin that I need.[9]

And Dennis Novack in his account of a dying patient, Adrienne, who was 'the first – and the last – patient to become my friend', emphasized dilemmas for the young physician.[10] 'I never again became so emotionally involved with a patient but, in the end, I was grateful for the experience. Adrienne deepened my understanding of patients' experiences of terminal illness and helped me overcome my fears of relating to these patients ... How do clinicians work out the conflicting emotions that sometimes arise.'

David Hilfiker's essay 'Clinical Detachment' is now well known for its explicit warning of the dangers of quelling one's emotional responses to patients:

> I had always been a rational, logical thinker; my emotional and intuitive side has always been underdeveloped – unfortunately true for many physicians; but the clinical detachment so necessary to medicine exacerbated such tendencies, encouraging them to emphasize them. Slowly, over the years the habit of dissociation became so ingrained in my personality that it invaded every nook and cranny of my life.[11]

Hilfiker goes on to say that he expected everyone around him to live the same way as a matter of course. 'It wasn't that I consciously valued that attitude toward life; but so powerful was its attraction, so difficult was it to switch out of it, that I found myself living with it more and more. What had begun as a technological tool became over the years a dominating force in my life.'

A subtle illustration appears in Milan Kunderer's *The Unbearable Lightness of Being* (noted in Chapter 2), in which clinical detachment appears to spill over into relationships with women and politics. In another novel, *The Case of Dr Sachs* by a physician-turned-writer, the issue comes down to a physician's choice not between two specialties or two styles of practice, but between two roles: doctor or care-giver. The author tells the reader that physicians are more comfortable as doctors: 'it looks better for parties and dinners, it looks better in the picture.'

The doctor 'knows', and his knowledge prevails over everything else. The care-giver seeks primarily to ease sufferings. The doctor expects patients and symptoms to fit the analytic format his school inculcated in him; the care-giver does his best (questioning his meagre certainties) to understand even slightly the things that happen to people. The doctor prescribes, the care-giver bandages. The doctor cultivates talk and power. The care-giver suffers.

As for the patient: no matter which he's dealing with, either way he's going to croak. But in what key?[12]

The overall advice, implicit if not explicit, from many such voices is that physicians must evaluate their responsibilities in relation to the emotional needs of their patients, and also recognise the negative and positive aspects of clinical detachment. It is often said that, generally speaking, this only happens after a physician's own serious illness, or by the impact of a single patient like Adrienne. As JA Katt wrote about another never-to-be-forgotten patient, Helen: 'She has changed the way I view patients. From her I learned that curing a disease is not always the most important aspect of the doctor–patient relationship ... Since Helen I treat all my patients with trust and respect, or try to, and perhaps more importantly, I treat them as equal human beings.'[13] Such introspection, it is argued, helps a physician to channel appropriate emotions into patient care – when it is warranted – as part of treatment, and to lessen the chances of being 'sucked' into, or caught unawares, in the web of emotional turmoil that can surround patients and their families.[14]

Medical education creates detachment

Medical education has been chastised for not addressing clinical detachment and the physician's need to be a person, at least in a consistent way. Physician David Loxterkamp, for instance, remarked that 'doctors are not trained to be tender. We are clinical commandos who target the chief complaint with skill, knowledge and the force of authority.' Loxterkamp was responding to a comment in the now classic book on a country doctor, *A Fortunate Man* (1967), by John Berger and Jean Mohr: 'the price of "facing, trying to understand, hoping to overcome the extreme anguish of other persons five or six times a week" was isolation, cyclical depression and eventual ruin.'[15]

Many observers see detachment not merely as an occupational hazard, but as an inevitable outcome of medical education. That the professionalisation (some say indoctrination) process of medical education 'hardens' or 'toughens' medical students, which in turn undermines such values as compassion, sensitivity and empathy, has long been noted. In the late eighteenth century, for instance, non-physician Thomas Gisborne warned every medical student about his 'heart [being] rendered hard, and his deportment unfeeling, by attendance on dissections of the dead and painful operations on the living.'[16] Much more recently, again in *A Fortunate Man* (1967), one can read that 'professional insulation' begins as medical students start dissecting the human body (cf. also Box 8.1).[17] Such sentiments open the door for such quips as 'Everyone else mourns the dead. Doctors cut them up.'[18]

Box 8.1   Medical students, human dissection and society

'You hear about those guys at Columbia?' said Harry. 'It was in the papers. They went to a subway change maker and when he gave them the token they put an amputated hand underneath the glass to pick it up. But as soon as he saw it the guy had a heart attack and died.' (Hafferty, 1991)

It is not easy to generalise about public attitudes toward medical students and human dissection, but mixed feelings and uneasiness certainly exist. Dissecting bodies – an early event in a medical student's education – is commonly seen as a key step in separating students from the general public. A substantial history of irreverent cartoons and photographs of students and cadavers goes hand in hand with the above cadaver story. There is, too, the story of Burke and Hare and their 'resurrection' of newly buried bodies from graveyards in Edinburgh during the 1820s to '30s; although now an historical vignette, it remains a generally well-known horror story, in part through a long line of feature films.

Anthropological studies such as FW Hafferty's *Into the Valley: death and the socialization of medical students* (1991) lend some support to concerns that students' anatomy experience encourages insensitivity. Hafferty's conclusions, from extended observations on a group of medical students, indicate that while some students maintain a human reference context for cadavers, others develop a 'biological' specimen or 'learning tool' perspective. The latter students, he indicates, must increase their tolerance of ambiguity in medicine if they are going to be receptive to the many equivocal and uncertain aspects of medical practice; they must continually examine their attitudes.

As one month dissolved into the next, the task of dissection acquired a certain routine. To dismember a body now seemed no more unnatural than to collect tolls on a highway or process bank loans.

Hafferty identified various stages in the anatomy experience of students when anxiety rose (and when bludgeoning might take place) as the student moved on to dissect parts of the body with particular cultural and symbolic meanings: 'If each time the cadaver raises its "humanistic" head the medical student beats it back with the bludgeon of scientific detachment, then we may expect that such a student will come to associate the reduction of situational stress with scientific distance and neutrality.'

The fact that, in many medical schools, students no longer dissect cadavers, but examine prosected body parts, may even reinforce insensitivity, for a sense may exist of examining pieces of meat without the context of face, hands and other characteristics that identify a person.

Anatomy is not viewed as the only culprit. It has been said that the early medical experiences of celebrated British psychiatrist RD Laing (1927–1989) 'were brutalising. [In] observing medical students and doctors toughening themselves against the distress of others, [Laing] began to criticise a system of medical care that distanced itself from the patients' pain and anxiety.'[19] Some talk of students learning to look upon patients as objects for study.[20] And surgeon Bernie Siegal said (1986):

> Although I do not believe that most physicians are villains, I do believe the training process is villainous. The student's natural desire to help people is drummed out of them by medical school training ... The prescribed attitude is called detached concern; however, such estrangement from your own feelings ultimately is deadly.[21]

Medical sociologists from the 1950s took increasing interest in the values and attitudes of medical students. Renée Fox, for instance, suggested that a difference between medical students of the 1950s and '70s was that the latter no longer admired the detached concern model;[22] however, the question remained: did, and does, disavowal of detachment in younger medical students necessarily persist? Does it mature into empathy with patients?[23] Many observers express doubts. In fact, the process of professionalisation in medical education continued to be viewed in the 1990s as 'traumatic de-idealisation', though one small study suggested that the cynicism and hostility that went with this was reduced among residents and even more so among faculty physicians.[24] Other studies have suggested that educational experience might inhibit moral reasoning ability rather than facilitating it.[25]

Whatever the impact of medical education – and certainly medical humanities/ ethics was playing a larger role by 2000 in trying to mitigate questionable professionalising forces – there is every reason to think that negative views of nascent doctors and of medical education (noted for its heavy emphasis on science to the virtual exclusion of the humanities) persist in the public mind. Such views are reinforced from various directions. For instance, media accounts of medical suicides such as three medical residents between October 1995 and January 1997 in Winnipeg, Canada.[26] Hollywood, too, raises many questionable images of medical students. In fact, its depictions of students, especially in a glut of movies in the late 1980s and early '90s often seen as reruns, painted a generally unflattering picture of their education; particularly noticeable are the stresses due to somewhat unfriendly institutions in which the students generally only have themselves for support (*see* Box 8.2).

Box 8.2   Hollywood and medical students: need for healing?

In the 1980s and early '90s, *Bad Medicine* (1985), *Gross Anatomy* (1989), *Vital Signs* (1990) and *Flatliners* (1990) all highlighted negative aspects of medical education. Aside from the anatomy scenes (almost horror scenes in *Flatliners*), the message – constantly reinforced by ready availability of the movies through videos and television reruns – is that the stress of medical school is hardly the best place for developing humane doctors.

Overwork was stressed In *Gross Anatomy* (1989), for instance, students were told:

> In the next eight months you will be required to memorize 6000 anatomical structures, read 25000 pages of text, attend 200 lectures and pass or fail 40 examinations. If you fail a class,

you have to repeat it. If you fail two, you have to repeat the entire term. If you fail three, well, let's just say, you probably don't belong here anyway ... Oh, by the way, the profession you just dedicated yourselves to carries with it the highest rate of alcoholism, drug addiction, divorce and suicide.

And in *Vital Signs*, third-year students heard:

Why would anyone knowingly do this to themselves? For the next year your days will not end, the work will never stop, your rank will command absolutely zero respect and worse of all, after it's over, you will be faced with the horrible realization that there is nothing in your medical career that will ever be as rewarding as third year. Third year is like being an 18-year-old rookie and being called to pitch the seventh game of the World Series – blindfolded!

Intense, unhealthy competition is made clear as students struggle to win the residency programmes of their choice. Tensions rise and drug abuse emerges. There is little time to socialise. A female student explains why she is not able to pursue a romantic interest: 'I have wanted to go to medical school ever since I can remember. This isn't a game for me. This has to be the most important thing right now. I'm just telling you this so you know why I have to work so hard, why I can't get distracted' (*Gross Anatomy*)

Medical student reviewers of the movies, at least up to the early 2000s, considered that, despite much embroidery, they had a strong basis in fact. Some observers, in noticing abuse and stress in medical schools, suggest there is a need for institutional healing if they are to produce humane doctors.

Amidst all this, there are always students, who, perhaps increasing in numbers with each new generation of students and with the help of medical humanities, do recognise the educational pitfalls and take corrective action. One student recounts how he relied on Samuel Shem's novel *The House of God* (1978) to remind him of what not to be: 'Every time I hear a joke about a patient or watch myself talk about what life will be like as a doctor, I think of it. I remind myself how much I don't want to become someone who contributes to the cycle of teaching medical students that *The House of God* is real – that patients, hospitals and medicine are the enemy.'[27]

A medical response

Physicians commonly recognise the pitfalls, both for patients and doctors, of detachment. Relatively few, however, suggest ways to balance emotional support for patients and the need to care for oneself as a person. Strikingly, the century-old teachings of William Osler remain relevant. In his now classic essay, 'Aequanimitas', delivered to medical students in 1889, Osler recommends the cultivation of imperturbability and equanimity (*see* Box 8.3). Although he did not mention these characteristics in the context of resolving the issue of clinical detachment and ensuring that one remains a person, this was implicit:

> Equanimity is chiefly exercised in enabling us to bear with composure the misfortunes of our neighbours. Now while nothing disturbs our mental placidity more sadly than straightened means, and the lack of those things after which the gentiles seek, I would warn you against the trials of the day soon to come to some of you – the day of large and successful practice. Engrossed late and soon in professional cares, getting and spending, you may so lay waste your powers that you find, too late, with hearts given away, that there is no place in your habit-stricken souls for those gentler influences which make life worth living.[28]

Box 8.3   The main points of Osler's essay, 'Aequanimitas'

1   Imperturbability (or coolness under fire and clear presence of mind)

- Remain cool with steady of hand under all circumstances.
- Control facial expressions; do not show anxiety or fear; without that, patients will lose confidence in you as their physician.
- Understand disease. This is the key to attaining imperturbability – the physician must know possible outcomes and know instantly what to do in all situations; imperturbability is partially heredity, but can be acquired through knowledge and experience.
- Imperturbability is often misinterpreted as hardness or apathy.
- Recognise that sensitivity is also important as long as it does not get in the way of one's coolness, or a surgeon's steadiness of hand.
- Find the balance between obtuseness to make firm, tough decisions and at the same time not losing the caring, loving side (hardening of the heart).

2   Equanimity (implying a fairness or justness of judgement and temperament, as well as poise and emotional balance)

- A calm equanimity is needed in all walks of life in our successes and our failures (cheerful equanimity).
- Natural temperament is involved, but one can still develop this calm equanimity.
- Don't expect too much from even your best patient; assume they will accept things from quack doctor reports such as cure-all medicines.
- Do not get angry with them for doing so. Accept it, as we have the same weaknesses as our patients.
- We need to have infinite patience with our patients.
- Equanimity will allow you to bear with composure other's misfortunes.
- But do not lose your caring side, as if that is let go, one may sacrifice the ability to enjoy many of the finer things of life.
- There is a great struggle ahead and it should be faced with a cheerful equanimity; even with imminent failure, we must keep our heads high and face it with a smile as opposed to 'crouching at its approach'.
- Patience is an equanimity allowing us to rise above the trials of life.

As with so much of Osler's writings his advice still resonates with the needs of today's physicians. Cultivating equanimity in a physician's practice has the potential to be less of a boundary-builder between patient and physician than consciously developing detachment. In fact, references to detachment in Osler's writings refer to separating oneself from 'the pursuits and pleasures incident to youth', and to being able to stand outside 'to take a philosophical view' of the profession as a whole.[29]

In spite of the persistent fame and continuing adulation of Osler, it has to be said that 'Aequanimitas' is little read today. This is not surprising if only because many physicians side-step the detachment issue.[30] Moreover, the medical profession's responses to the role of physician as a person tend to focus on treating major problems associated with substance abuse with perhaps less attention being given to preventing stress or burn-out. Calls for medical education to help develop skills in lifelong coping strategies are generally only partially met in curricula, yet one wonders whether this could have helped the dilemmas of one doctor with allegiances both to her non-physician husband and to medicine as described in her story 'Marrying Medicine'.[31] Stress or wellness programmes, in dealing with the rigours and perils of professional life, might point up the potential role – suitable for at least some practitioners – of the humanities in stress management, a point generally left out of otherwise sound advice (cf. Box 8.4). Physician poets, such as John Stone, often emphasise that writing poetry can contribute to one becoming a better physician and that poetry has the power to heal.[32]

Box 8.4   How do people become reflective practitioners? A reflective questioning technique

Use of self

- What is my role within this situation? What is the patient's role?
- How does my role interface with the patient's role? With other people's roles in this setting?
- What personal qualities do I bring to this interaction?
- What are my personal biases and assumptions? How might these assumptions be helpful? A hindrance?
- How can I balance my professional role with the ultimate experience of being human?

Knowledge and expertise

- How has my training prepared me for working with this person (or within this setting)? What previously acquired knowledge and skills can I apply? What knowledge and skills do I need to learn?
- What specific theories would help me to better understand this person?

Problem setting

- How am I framing the problem that I am trying to solve? What are my goals for this patient? For myself?
- How might this problem be viewed from a patient's perspective?

- What are the patient's goals?
- What issues are being expressed?
- What do I need to know about this person to better understand his/her perspective?
- How might this problem be viewed from the family's perspective? From the perspective of other team members?

Strategies

- What specific strategies might be helpful in this situation?
- What strategies have I tried? Which have been successful? Unsuccessful?
- What other strategies might I consider trying?

Learning from experience

- How has my involvement with this person changed my practice?
- How am I a different person because of this experience?
- What will I do differently the next time?

(From Sekulic A and Nekolaischuk C (1998) Being Well. *Bulletin of the Society of Professional Well-being.* **10** (2): 7.)

Physicians who talk about how they cope with the daily grind invariably demonstrate the importance of reflection as does physician–writer David Loxtercamp in his homily on the moral virtues of practising rural medicine. He is one who believes virtue must be looked for in every 'walk of life'. For him, as he works in what many see as the humdrum side of medicine, a country practice: 'virtue is about the everyday responsibility of living in a community. It is not the province of heroes or saints whom we idolize and elevate and leave holding the bag. We must overcome fear and modesty in order to reclaim virtue and a fuller sense of ourselves.'[33]

Reflections: know thyself

Reflection on one's own practices can be difficult for many people. David Hilfiker points out that doctors will not admit that 'perfection is a grand illusion' – 'a game of mirrors that everyone plays.' One reason, he says, is that 'doctors hide their mistakes from patients, from other doctors, even from themselves. Open discussion of mistakes is banished from the consultation room, from the operating room, from physicians' meetings ... Unable to admit our mistakes, we physicians are cut off from healing. We cannot ask for forgiveness, and we get none. We are thwarted, stunted; we do not grow.'[34] Although this fits the quip that 'MD' is an abbreviation for 'massive denial', it has to be said that the early twenty-first century is witnessing significant efforts to ensure a changed attitude towards medical mistakes, such that lessons can be learned by the profession, healthcare administrators and the public.[35]

Does a game of mirrors – Hilfiker's phrase – always centre on illusions? Countless artists have shown that looking into mirrors offers a thought-provoking way to reflect on ourselves, even on our other beings. For instance, to see a subversive 'double', or *doppelganger*, in ourselves, albeit much less hidden than in, for instance, Robert Louis Stevenson's classic story of the vicious Mr Hyde and the virtuous Dr Jekyll.[36] The artist can prompt reflection in many other ways. One is about our mortality. It is often said that, notwithstanding the ever presence of death in medical practice, physicians only become sensitive to mortality and its meaning for patients after their own serious illness. Perhaps it is not surprising that, although medical education has been paying formal attention since the 1970s to the diversity of sensitivities and meanings attached to death, this still receives relatively little attention in most curricula. One picture, an important resource in medical humanities, especially for students studying anatomy, is Rembrandt's masterpiece, 'Anatomy of Dr Nicolaes Tulp' (1632). As one of the best known paintings in medical history, it offers many points for discussion, particularly for medical students facing anatomy for the first time with, as said, its potential for fostering detachment.

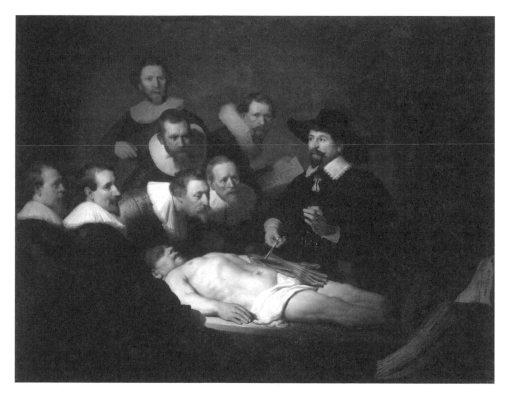

Figure 8.1 Rembrandt's 'Anatomy of Dr Nicolaes Tulp' (1632). Canvas, 169.5 × 216.5 cm.
Source: The Royal Picture Gallery, Mauritshuis, The Hague. Reproduced with permission.

Art historians and others have long debated many aspects of the picture (*see* Figure 8.1). Aside from interest in identifying the observers in the picture – all Amsterdam surgeons – two interpretations of the picture prompt comment here.[37]

1 *As an anatomy picture*. A question commonly asked is whether Rembrandt depicted an accurate anatomical lesson in the muscles in the forearm. The most recent comprehensive study confirms that it is a demonstration of the muscles flexing the fingers of the hand. Tulp holds in his forceps the flexor digitorum superficialis muscle away from the flexor digitorum profundus muscle, which is a long straight muscle running underneath it. By lifting the superficialis away from the profundus, he reveals the way in which the two muscles combine their strength to flex the fingers.

An important issue is whether Rembrandt chose the hand as a theme for any particular reason. Seemingly the choice was in line with a long history of seeing the complexity of hand movements – far different from the claws or hooves of animals – as pointing to the creation of human civilisation that raised men above the animal kingdom. Thus, in one way, Tulp was not only illustrating the anatomy of the body, but also illuminating the presence of God in man.

2 *A picture with an enduring theme*. A further interpretation of the painting, calling on a knowledge of the real life of Tulp and his anatomical knowledge, is that it raises a basic issue, a dichotomy, in thinking about the ancient proverb 'Know thyself'. The dichotomy hinges on two views: (1) the divinity and immortality of the human being, and (2) the mortality and ephemeral nature of humans.

While other surgeons of Tulp's time pointed out the mortality of man, Tulp was predisposed to the existence of an elusive metaphysical element that does not die. In Rembrandt's time, discussion existed on how anatomy illustrates the manifestation of God in the human body. This, in the words of sixteenth- and seventeenth-century anatomists, was to 'know thyself'.

Of special interest is the change in the attitudes towards anatomy since the time of Tulp and Rembrandt. Although anatomy education had practical purposes by the sixteenth and seventeenth centuries (e.g. for surgery), anatomies were, unlike nowadays, also linked to the search for self-knowledge, to the exploration of such matters as one's place in nature, to understanding the source of passions and how to conquer them, and to the reality of mortality.

Appendix: 'The Woody Allen Report on Physicians'[38]

Countless other resources from the humanities can prompt reflection on the doctor as a person, and on his or her position in society. This chapter ends with notes on the movies of Woody Allen. Placed as an appendix because it is far removed from the 'serious' art of Rembrandt, it nevertheless offers an interesting mirror of medical practice, especially in how to respond (or not respond) to what are often viewed as 'difficult' patients.

Woody Allen, acknowledged as one of the most influential, critiqued and studied modern filmmakers, who has remained relatively non-Hollywood and non-commercial, is an acknowledged commentator on contemporary society.[39] Allen examines and challenges a largely urbanised, industrialised, technologically dependent and institutionalised modern society. Additionally, he has paid special attention over many years to the medical profession.

In countless vignettes Allen depicts a patient's experience with physicians as he offers critical, albeit invariably satirical, images of physicians. His overall views of physicians can best be understood as from a composite patient compiled from various characters in his films. Although the patient might be described as a narcissistic hypochondriac, we see an individual struggling in a modern society, an individual with commonplace fears, needs and expectations. Thus, Allen presents a character with human shortcomings, albeit with a self-awareness of them. He deals openly with subjects which are commonly uncomfortable, such as the fear of death and loss of control over one's life due to physical and mental illness.

Allen first asks the question, what do patients expect when they go to the doctor? If the primary concerns of the patient are not met, what are the issues arising from the failed interaction? In asking these questions, Allen underscores a series of issues, many ethical, which have become increasingly vexing in recent years, especially physician–patient relationships and the dominant authority of the physician. Behind all topics, Allen constantly asks, what are the patient's rights? His patient expects a physician to respect his autonomy, to have sensitivity, and needs to be able to trust the physician's professional expertise and conduct. The patient wants healing in the whole sense, to walk away from the experience with mental and emotional comfort. The order of priority of a patient's needs and expectations change from film to film and Allen is asking for each situation to be examined on its own merits.

It should be noted that *Crimes and Misdemeanors* is one film with an exception to Allen's general imagery of physicians. In this case, the representation of the physician is not from the experience of the patient, but from a more in-depth study of the physician as a person. By shifting the narrative to focus on the physician, Allen creates a character who comes across to his patients as a 'good' physician; unnervingly, however, patients are unable to see the dark side.

Illustrative films to 1990

What's New, Pussycat? (1965)

What's New, Pussycat? is Allen's first screenplay. It is about a womaniser who seeks help from a psychiatrist so that he can settle down with the woman he loves. Upon arriving at his first session, the patient sees the psychiatrist throwing a temper tantrum at his wife; later the psychiatrist trades places with the patient on the couch and admits to his uncontrollable lust for a female patient. Throughout the film there is a constant shifting of roles, while we see the psychiatrist's sexual misconduct and violation of every ethical code. Allen plays a secondary character in the film and, although not in the role of a patient, talks the psychiatrist out of wrapping himself in the French flag and setting fire to himself.

Everything You Always Wanted To Know About Sex* (*but were afraid to ask) (1972)

This is a satire on a celebrated book on sex written by physician David Reuben in 1969. Although on one level the book presents itself as free and liberated by openly discussing sexuality, it assumes a rather dogmatic, expert-oriented approach to sexuality. Allen's film is a series of vignettes on subjects addressed by the book, including aphrodisiacs, sodomy, perversion, transvestites, homosexuality and biomedical research on human sexuality. One vignette, on sodomy, depicts a patient, who is in love with a sheep, consulting a general practitioner. The physician is floored and cannot respond. However, eventually the physician himself falls in love with the sheep, becoming 'crazy', as he had called the patient.

Another vignette on biomedical research on sexuality shows two unwilling patients trapped by an insane, highly published doctor in his laboratory where he is conducting horrific experiments on non-consenting human subjects. When confronted with the idea of ethics, he responds by calling it 'nonsense', saying the research will make him rich.

Sleeper (1973)

Here, the patient, an innocent victim of modern science, entered hospital for routine peptic ulcer surgery, only to face complications and be cryogenically frozen (without consent). On waking up 200 years in the future, he is manipulated by other physicians. We see the patient's profound lack of confidence in the professional expertise, ethical conduct and degree of uncertainty amongst doctors. The patient sees them as only self-interested, power-minded and unqualified.

Annie Hall (1977)

This film focuses on the experience of a patient with a Freudian-trained psychoanalyst. The patient is caught in a cycle of dependence and dissatisfaction with psychoanalysis, being hopelessly dependent on the therapy, not believing in its validity, and holding a complete lack of trust in the professional expertise and character of the doctor. Moreover, he feels the doctor's lack of respect for his autonomy, as well as the unequal power relationship between them. This disempowers the patient, leaving his life to be controlled by the doctor. Despite 15 years of psychoanalysis, five times a week – which has made the doctor rich – his problems persist, albeit eased by taking Valium.

Manhattan (1979)

Allen's patient is further disillusioned with doctors when he experiences one with extreme 'unorthodox' methods. On one hand, there is a strict Freudian who maintains an authoritarian stance with the patient, and then there is Donny, a non-traditional analyst who calls his patient up in the middle of the night and weeps, and eventually has a drug-induced nervous breakdown. The 'farce' that doctors are omnipotent and infallible to human shortcomings is played out.

Stardust Memories (1980)

The patient encounters more uncaring, self-oriented, incompetent doctors. One who takes blood pressure in the middle of a chaotic business meeting with screaming all around, then hands the patient a packet of Valium. The other an authoritarian, ambitious academic who didn't help the patient, but named a disorder after him for publication and speeches at conferences.

Zelig (1983)

This film demonstrates the patient's experience with his ethical rights being completely violated, and the delicate nature of the roles, dynamics and boundaries in the relationship with the physician. Zelig, who is just like anyone in that he wants love and acceptance, finds that he is healed by violating every traditional guideline in the physician–patient relationship. When his first attempt at gaining equal stature with his doctor – by insisting that he is a doctor – fails, he finds that he is still treated with respect by a woman doctor. He starts to trust this doctor, eventually falling in love with her, and she reciprocates. It is ironic that engaging in ethical misconduct and developing a personal relationship is the only thing which cures the patient. Allen, like others, believes that boundaries are questionable.

The film also prompts the question, what (or who) is normal?

Hannah and Her Sisters (1986)

Mickey Rose is a self-admitted hypochondriac, and acknowledges how he may be a difficult patient. The physicians he encounters, however, deliberately seem to ignore his problem, and, even in the face of his worries, seem to grow colder in manner. First, he encounters a doctor who coldly reports his infertility and states that it has been known to destroy many healthy relationships. He then has an experience in which his worst fear as a hypochondriac may come true – he may have something seriously wrong with him. His doctor, knowing his fears, doesn't even talk to him face to face in the same room, and coldly says that he doesn't like the results of the hearing test and would like a series of high-tech tests run at the hospital. Calling another one of his many doctors he is told over the phone it could be a brain tumour. The patient experiences the magnitude of power found in information, especially when used carelessly.

Crimes and Misdemeanors (1989)

This film is the exception to the general physician images in Allen's films in that it is a character study of the physician. It is evident from this film that Allen's long history of negative experiences with the medical profession has led him to believe physicians can be devoid of any moral structure – up to the point of being a borderline sociopath. The physician here is aware of his nature, and goes through a learning process by discovering gradually that he is capable of great evil, without remorse. He accepts this about himself, and lives on to prosper, literally getting away with murder. In this sense the patient has realised that physicians are fallible, subject to the whole of human nature, including the darker aspects.

Alice (1990)

Frustrated with the negative experiences and lack of healing from the medical profession's 'traditional' western side, and amidst a crisis, the patient tries an alternative form of healing from a doctor of Chinese medicine, Dr Yang. Although not evident at first, this turns out to be the right move for the patient. Dr Yang provides respect for the patient's autonomy and listens well. The patient expects to receive some sort of herbal treatments or acupuncture, but the sessions wind up more as psychotherapy. After getting the patient to talk about emotional distress, the focus is taken away from the physical problems, although Dr Yang gives the patient 'special' herbs at the end of each visit. These herbs always do magical things, yet seem to be a placebo meant to satisfy the patient's expectation for a 'magic bullet'. The patient initially ignores the psychoemotional aspects of Dr Yang's treatment, focusing on the physical effects of the herbs; however, by the end of the experience with Dr Yang she realises the herbs are irrelevant to the problem and are not necessary, and she has gone through a process of healing in a whole sense. It is then that the patient's endless search through the medical profession ends, no longer expecting an absolute answer from science, or detaching the physician from the human being.

Endnotes

1   Broyard A (1992) The patient examines the doctor. In: Broyard A *Intoxicated By My Illness and Other Writings on Life and Death*. Clarkson Potter, New York, p. 44.

2   Nowadays, with more and more women entering medicine, this expression is out of date, and is perhaps best expressed as a 'jealous paramour'.

3   Center for Professional Well-Being, Durham, North Carolina founded by John-Henry Pfifferling PhD.

4   Lipsky E (1972) *Malpractice*. William Morrow, New York, p. 7. Dans PE (2000) *Doctors in the Movies. Boil the Water and Just Say Aah*. Medi-Ed Press, Bloomington, pp. 288–9 notes that similar emphases on long hours is a recurring theme in movies. For instance, *No Way Out* (1950) includes a hospital doctor arriving home weary after caring for the injured in a race riot; his maid says to him, 'You can use a day off.' He replies, 'I had one once.'

5   Cook R (1972) *The Year of the Intern*. Harcourt Brace Jovanovich, New York, p. 4.

6   Gash J (1998) *Prey Dancing*. Penguin Books, New York, p. 8.

7   Linzer M (1994) Blueberry muffins and mystery novels. *Annals of Internal Medicine*. **121**: 56–7.

8   Some points are made by Kim J (2001) Emotional detachment and involvement of physicians in literature. *The Pharos*. **64**: 32–8.

9   Selzer R (1979) An absence of wisdom. In his *Confessions of a Knife*. Simon and Schuster, New York, p. 18.

10 Novack DH (1993) Adrienne. *Annals of Internal Medicine*. **119**: 424–5.

11 Hilfiker D (1998) Clinical detachment. In his *Healing the Wounds: a physician looks at his work*. Creighton University Press, Omaha, pp. 100–1.

12 Winckler M (2000) *The Case of Dr Sachs*. Seven Stories, New York, pp. 384–5.

13 Katt JA (1992) Core curriculum. *Annals of Internal Medicine*. **117**: 607.

14 One illustration of being caught in the web of family emotions and needs can be found in Barnard D (1986) A case of amyotrophic lateral sclerosis. *Literature and Medicine*. **5**: 27–42. This is a narrative by a participant observer of a physician and her relations with an elderly patient suffering from the disease, and with the patient's wife increasingly burdened as care-giver. The purpose of the narrative is to depict 'illness as a shared experience in the lives of sufferer and healer'. The article and its analysis attracted much attention. See commentaries by Rabkin E (1986) A case of self-defense, ibid., pp. 43–53, and Smith D (1986) The limits of narratives, ibid., pp. 54–7.

15 Loxterkamp D (1999) Facing our morality: the virtue of a common life. *Journal of the American Medical Association*. **282**: 923–4.

16 Quoted from Porter R (1993) Thomas Gisborne: physicians, christians, and gentlemen. In: Wear A, Geyer-Kordesh J and French R (eds) *Doctors and Ethics: the earlier historical setting of professional ethics*. Rodopi, Amsterdam, p. 257.

17 Berger J and Mohr J (1967) *A Fortunate Man: the story of a country doctor*. Allen Lane, London, p. 105.

18 Quoted from Winckler (2000) *The Case of Dr Sachs*, p. 384.

19 Stewart H (1996) Glasgow's doomed visionary. *Guardian Weekly*. August 11, p. 29.

20 Inlander CB, Levin LS and Weiner E (1988) *Medicine on Trial: the appalling story of ineptitude, malfeasance, neglect and arrogance*. Prentice Hall, New York, p. 86.

21   Quoted in Borins M (1991) Current events. Bernie Siegal: peace, love and healing. *Humane Medicine.* **7** (2): 129–32.

22   Compare a paper written by Fox in the mid-1950s, The autopsy: attitude-learning of second-year medical students, eventually published in Fox RC (1979) *Essays in Medical Sociology: journeys into the field.* Wiley & Sons, New York, pp. 51–77, along with Is there a 'new' medical student?: a comparative view of medical socialization in the 1950s and the 1970s, reprinted in ibid., pp. 78–101.

23   The existence of debates on whether empathy can be taught was noted in Chapter 4. In relation to the writings of Fox, see also Spiro H (1992) What is empathy and can it be taught? *Annals of Internal Medicine.* **116**: 843–6.

24   See Testerman JK, Morton KR, Loo LK *et al.* (1996) The natural history of cynicism in physicians. *Academic Medicine.* **71** (10 supplement): S43–S45.

25   Self DJ, Schrader DE, De Baldwin DeWC and Wolinsky FD (1991) A pilot study of the relationship of medical education and moral development. [abstract]. *Academic Medicine.* **66**: 629. Yet a further investigation indicated a *decline* of ethical sensitivities in the third and fourth years in the University of Toronto, and elsewhere, and of the 'erosion' of ethical principles: Hébert PC, Meslin EM and Dunn EV (1992) Measuring the ethical sensitivity of medical students: a study at the University of Toronto. *Journal of Medical Ethics.* **18**: 142–7. See also Feudtner C, Christakis DA and Christakis NA (1994) Do clinical clerks suffer ethical erosion? Students' perceptions of their ethical environment and personal development. *Academic Medicine.* **69**: 670–9.

26   It is indicative of rising concerns among young physicians that the Manitoba Medical Student's Association responded to the suicides by publishing what they saw as stress factors that included large student debt loads; being forced to choose a field of special-isation in the third year of medical school; government limitations in connection with place of practice; long hours, which cause strain and breakdown of relationships; reduced number of resident positions, as a result of cutbacks, with more work for each resident; reduced quality of patient care when sleep-deprived, and frequent examinations requiring large amounts of studying and research. Additionally noted were the stresses inherent in the everyday practice of medicine: ambiguity/ambivalence and uncertainty surrounding much clinical practice, the contrast between the orderly approach of 'rational' scientific knowledge and the indeterminacy of patients. See Williams LS (1997) Manitoba suicides force consideration of stresses facing medical residents. *Canadian Medical Association Journal.* **156**: 1599–602.

27   The House of God. *Student BMJ* 2002; **10**: 481; www.studentbmj.com/back_issues/1202/reviews/481.html (accessed July 2004). It is of interest to include here further quotes from Justin Denholm. '*The House of God* has been hanging over my head from the beginning. When I was accepted into medicine, I was given a copy by a helpful fourth year student who told me that I had to read it to understand "what medicine is really like". So I read it before ever sitting in a lecture, trailing after a ward round, or touching a patient.' Denholm adds that the book stunned him, but he convinced himself that it simply wasn't true. 'I put the book away and got on with becoming a doctor.' However, during his last two years in medical school, *The House of God* became his Sword of Damocles. 'Every time I hear a joke about a patient or watch myself talk about what life will be like as a doctor, I think of it. I remind myself how much I don't want to become someone who contributes to the cycle of teaching medical students that the *The House of God* is real – that patients, hospitals and medicine are the enemy.'

28   Quoted from reprint in Roland C (ed) (1982) *Sir William Osler 1849–1919: a selection for medical students.* The Hannah Institute for the History of Medicine, Toronto, p. 5.

29   Quoted in Camac CNB (1905) *Counsels and Ideals from the Writings of William Osler.* Houghton Mifflin, Boston, p. 86 (reprint, Birmingham: The Classics of Medicine Library, 1985) and Silverman ME, Murray TJ and Bryan CS (eds) (2003) *The Quotable Osler.* American College of Physicians, Philadelphia, p. 17.

30   One says this in spite of the fact that, for many years, all Canadian students have received a copy of the essay, distributed by Associated Medical Services, Ontario. In: Roland (1982) *Sir William Osler.*

31   Van Peenan HJ (2000) Marrying medicine. In: LaCombe M (ed) *On Being a Doctor 2.* American College of Physicians, Philadelphia, pp. 133–9.

32 John Stone, Professor of Medicine (Cardiology), Emeritus, at Emory University School of Medicine, has published five books of poetry. His essays relevant to medical humanities are collected in *In the Country of Hearts: journeys in the art of medicine* (1996) Louisiana State University Press, Baton Rouge.

33 Loxterkamp D (1999) Facing our morality: the virtue of a common life. *Journal of the American Medical Association.* **282**: 923–4.

34 In Hilfiker (1998) *Healing the Wounds*, p. 59.

35 Much emphasis is now being placed on medical errors, including system errors. One index of this is over two million hits on Google for 'medical errors', July 2004.

36 Miller J (1998) *On Reflection*. National Gallery Publications, London, considers in this mind-expanding book the many artists who have incorporated and interpreted mirror images in their paintings.

37 The discussion here rests on Shupbach W (1982) The paradox of Rembrandt's 'Anatomy of Dr Tulp'. *Medical History* Supplement 2, Wellcome Institute for the History of Medicine, London.

38 This appendix draws on an unpublished study undertaken by a medical student, David Pitchon.

39 The literature on Allen is substantial. A still useful discussion that centres on his early films, mostly discussed here, is Shapiro B (1986) Woody Allen's search for self. *Journal of Popular Culture.* **19** (4): 47–62.

Part 2

Physician as clinical decision maker: public voices, metaphors and stereotypes

Part 1 has focused on roles and issues that primarily impinge on humane care in clinical practice. In contrast, the public's wish for one of the physician's roles to be a clinical decision maker (in the original EFPO surveys this was coupled with 'medical expert') draws particular attention to a practitioner's medical knowledge and skills. One aspect of this is a wish to be able to assess, or at least to have a better sense of, their doctor's 'up-to-dateness'. A difficult question for any lay person is who would they choose, *if they had to*, between either a young doctor with extensive clinical knowledge but who shows little thought for a patient's feelings, or an elderly doctor with untold empathy but who is suspected of being out of date.

For many people, judging their physicians depends not only on successful outcomes, but also on whether the practitioner is a good expositor of medical science for which communication skills are as important as factual knowledge, a point noted in Chapter 5. Also noted earlier is that communication skills are dependent on more than a detailed knowledge of facts. One consideration is that a patient's interpretation of 'facts' may be different from the physician's due to particular needs and attitudes towards illness, and different approaches to interpreting information.

Part 2, with further perspectives from the humanities, especially history, points to various factors that can shape a physician's interpretation of 'facts', or at least shape the use of those facts in ways that affect clinical decision making. Particular attention is given to metaphors and stereotypes (Chapters 9 and 10) and to concepts of disease (Chapter 11).

CHAPTER 9

Clinical decisions

The good doctor and diagnostic skills

The public has long identified diagnostic skills as a mark of the 'good' physician. Examples of diagnostic prowess and triumphs are readily found in popular culture. Dr Leonard Gillespie, the wise and crusty physician in the popular Dr Kildare movies from 1937 to 1947 (*see also* Chapter 2), was the consummate diagnostician. And, in the 1945 novel *Medical Practice*, the death of a fiancée due to a 'wrong diagnosis' led physician Peter McDonald to become a 'diagnostician' instead of following in his father's footsteps into general practice.[1] In fact, the public esteem given to diagnosis – partly due to reverence for the latest medical science and technology – was one factor behind the rising status, from the 1920s onward, of specialists over general medical practitioners. In 1930, one American physician opined that the 'latest substitute for the breadth of vision of the general practitioner is that offspring of the American God of Efficiency, the Diagnostic Clinic'. He added that such clinics, owned by groups of specialists, were sometimes run as machines where 'the patient is automatically passed from one specialist to another ... submitted to a series of examinations, so detailed in their nature that it would seem that nothing could be overlooked', and with no one practitioner there to 'understand the situation as a whole'.[2]

Such sentiments can still be heard today, just as the esteem placed on diagnostic prowess remains high; indeed, being a 'diagnostician' in any occupation carries the caché of expertise. In the United States it is not uncommon to find internists advertising their skills as diagnosticians.[3] Moreover, the eminent diagnostician continues to be found in novels. *The Cunning Man* (1994), for instance, is written as the memoirs (from World War II onwards) of a Toronto physician, who is revealed as a highly regarded, if unorthodox, diagnostician.[4]

It is not surprising that the physician and eminent novelist Walker Percy (1916–1990) elected to pursue the theme of diagnosis through much of his literary work. He said that the expertise of the 'physician–novelist is not in the business of writing edifying tales', but 'in the business of *diagnosis*, not therapy' of social ills.[5] On another occasion, Percy said: 'I'm trying to be a diagnostician who makes a little sense out of a malaise, a disease, or rather a dis-ease that influences our lives more than we care to – dare to – realize, or admit to ourselves, never mind anyone else.'[6]

Percy's phrase, the 'business of diagnosis', prompts thoughts about medical and social pressures for *exact* diagnoses. Aside from concepts of specificity that, today, drive both drug research and drug marketing, administrators and governments want statistics on diagnostic categories in order to make policy decisions.[7] Patients, too, often search for a diagnosis that satisfies them; this has contributed to increasing numbers of people, particularly since the 1980s, looking outside conventional medicine towards alternative medicine. In his usual satirical way, Woody Allen (*see* appendix to Chapter 8) captured a sense of this in his 1990 movie, *Alice*. A bored housewife, Alice was not only worried about chemicals in food, but also about her back problem for which she had tried many practitioners including chiropractic and massage. A friend told her about 'a brilliant diagnostician':

> Dr Yang is not just an acupuncturist, he's a brilliant diagnostician. And he gives these herbs; the man's a genius. He diagnoses you from your pulse. He took Jean Lewis's pulse and told her she was going to develop an ulcer. No western doctor could find it ... Six months later she fell over with pain ... His herbs are marvellous; they're not chemicals, they're all natural substances.

It turned out that Dr Yang, a doctor of traditional Chinese medicine, did not diagnose a back problem in Alice, but something in the 'mind' and the 'heart', a diagnosis that led to a transformation in her empty life.[8]

Satisfying patients

> It has been said that one person in five suffers from inactivity of the large bowel or colon. Though there may be more or less movement of the bowels the colon is sluggish and waste material remains there to poison the blood and give rise to tired, languid feelings as well as keen suffering from such painful ailments as rheumatism and lumbago. The teeth and tonsils are often blamed for poisons which originate in the colon. (1936 Almanac)[9]

> A bad acidosis he had said to Sanders earlier in the evening, and his diagnosis had been confirmed. Orange juice, glucose, the regulation treatment ... [It] had resulted from some deficiency or diet or a general condition. (Physician' comment in 1940 novel)[10]

A diagnosis needs to satisfy both patients and medical colleagues. Satisfying patients can be the most challenging, especially if the explanation for the condition fails to embrace all of a patient's symptoms, or the physician does not recognise and take into account a patient's own belief systems and understanding of disease.

Clashes between conventional and lay medical diagnoses have a long history. Those expressed in the two quotations that open this section – autointoxication due to inadequate removal of poisons from the gut, and acidosis or excess acid in the blood (both accepted by many physicians during the first half of the twentieth century) – have been rejuvenated in recent years in popular, not professional, health books and articles. Moreover, medical issues surrounding lay diagnoses were increasingly highlighted during the last decades of the twentieth century with the growth of multiculturalism in western societies.[11] Ethnic issues have been voiced in many ways. Particularly noticeable are aboriginal beliefs captured imaginatively in, for example, many novels such as *Bad Medicine* (1998), already noted in Chapter 7. The latter centres on a rare outbreak of the little known Hanta virus among Navaho people in the South-Western United States. The novel's concerns and questions about the adequacy of scientific explanations to satisfy many cultural sensitivities clearly challenge many conventional wisdoms.[12]

Although both physicians and lay people may seem to attach greater respect to diagnostic skills than to therapy – the latter is given relatively little formal attention (e.g. as courses) in medical schools – a note on therapy is necessary if only because it is an issue in public perceptions of up-to-dateness. Patients are naturally concerned with finding successful treatments, and, over time, many doctors have developed a 'special' reputation for their 'medicines'. However, as the pharmaceutical industry became more powerful and the use of standardised, manufactured prescription medications had become the norm by around the 1950s (rather than pharmacists compounding medicines from multiple constituents prescribed for individual patients), the 'art' of therapy diminished during the second half of the twentieth century. More standardised approaches based on information from the promotional literature and the representatives of the pharmaceutical industry, from textbooks, and from guidelines established by 'experts' became even more evident. Many patients now voice doubts whether their medical treatment is tailored to their individual needs such as gender, weight, metabolism, etc. The view that the doctor treats the disease and not the patient constantly hovers.[13]

Any detailed look at popular and professional concepts of, and attitudes towards, disease follows many directions. While many are inappropriate to pursue for this volume, comments are appropriate on the role of metaphors and stereotypes, which, as the humanities make clear, permeate our culture. Although the precise impact on clinical decision of metaphors and stereotypes is conjectural, they, as will be illustrated, can be issues in, for instance, infectious diseases, cancer, neurology, psychiatry, gender and health, and the heart and cardiology. Above all, the war on disease metaphor is strikingly pervasive as we now explore.

Metaphors and clinical decision making: war on disease

In the past 30 years or so, ever since Susan Sontag's influential book *Illness as Metaphor* (1978) critiqued the place of metaphors in healthcare, attention has been given to their frequency and role.[14] Countless examples exist, covering, for example, how the body works ('the body is like an engine'), medicine is like detective work ('cracking the genetic code'), and in the healthcare system 'health is a commodity'. By far the largest number of metaphors, however, centre on warfare ('an attack of measles', 'she lost the battle with cancer', 'the immune system fights infection', 'ideal drugs are magic bullets', and so on). Sontag argues that such metaphors mystify and can stigmatise disease, and hence should be stripped from healthcare. Nevertheless, the comments in the rest of this chapter suggest that this is not only an impractical proposition, but would also undermine coping mechanisms for many patients.

> Perpetual warfare ought to be waged against those who wilfully cough and sneeze into the open without protecting the face with a handkerchief. (1917)[15]
>
> Today we are sending you out to battle. Only you are not armed with poison gas and bayonets, but with antiseptic, chloroform and healing hands. For you march not in the path of Alexander and Napoleon, but of Semmelweis, Lister and Pasteur. Fight your war with courage and honesty, young men, for yours is a war against death. (1941)[16]

> When an oncologist was asked recently (2002) 'What is it like losing a patient?' he replied, 'You don't lose the patient, you lose the battle with disease.' 'Cancer', he claimed, 'is my enemy, and as an oncologist it is my job to eradicate this enemy.'[17]

The sense of war against disease is part of a long history of the use of war metaphors in medicine. Although they are most common with infectious diseases and cancers, they extend to countless other conditions. An important issue, as indicated, is whether a mindset of 'war on disease' has implications for everyday medical practice. For instance, does it unconsciously lead some practitioners to be more interventionist than others in using diagnostic tests, and more vigorous in their treatments, either surgical or medical? Perhaps, too, it tends to focus attention on the disease to the exclusion of the person. Does it contribute to doctors being divided into 'do-ers', who aggressively attack the source of the difficulty, and 'watchers', who see how much the body can do for itself and consider that the role of the physician is to give it a helpful nudge now and then?[18] Such a dichotomy – long-standing among physicians – can reflect the extent to which a practitioner sees him or herself as aiding 'natural' healing powers (or trusting the healing power of nature).

The concept of natural healing power – often referred to as *vis medicatrix naturae* – deserves comment here since it sharpens our appreciation of the mindset of *fighting* disease by offering an alternative approach. The concept of the healing power of nature has a long history of waxing and waning in popularity in conventional medicine, and has a reciprocal relationship with the rise and fall of interventionist treatment that reflects an 'attack' mode. A notable example of the latter is 'heroic' therapy – characterised by, for example, the administration of large doses of medicaments – that was especially evident during the first half of the nineteenth century. When Oliver Wendell Holmes opposed heroic regimens in 1860, he indicated he was siding with what was then a 'heresy' of trusting nature, while offering nature help.[19] Generally speaking, since the early decades of the twentieth century the overall trend in conventional medicine has not been to trust nature. An indicator of this, especially since World War II, is the general acceptance of powerful drugs, invasive tests and complex surgery.[20]

Despite this trend, the concept of natural healing acquired increasing vigour during the last decades of the twentieth century. This was largely through the growing popularity of complementary and alternative medicine in which various practitioners were seen to have 'healing power' by marshalling the powers of nature and the healing powers of the body. Such notions often meld into the themes of magic and healing widely circulated in our culture through novels and movies ranging from the phenomenally successful Harry Potter stories (for instance, the healing powers of Madame Pomfrey, the Hogwart's 'school nurse') to the movie *The Green Mile* (1999) in which a wrongly accused death row inmate reveals powers of faith healing.

Amid the growth of lay interest in the healing power of nature, some contemporary physicians see it as central to their practice; as one wrote in a book directed to lay and professional audiences (1997):

> But always the purpose of treatment is only to restore nature's balance against disease. There is no recovery unless it comes from the force and fibre of one's own tissues. The physician's role is to be

the cornerman – stitch up the lacerations, apply the soothing balm, encourage the fighter's specific abilities, say all the right things – to encourage the flagging strength of the real combatant, the pummelled body. As doctors, we do our best when we remove the obstacles to healing and encourage organs and cells to use their own nature-given power to overcome.[21]

Practitioners who pay little attention to this concept of natural healing, or see it as relatively ineffective, are more likely to hold the 'war on disease' mindset. This mindset began to become more evident in the early twentieth century in the wake of the germ theory of disease, and especially with the work of Paul Ehrlich (1854–1915).[22] Salvarsan, his newly discovered chemical treatment for syphilis (introduced 1910), along with the emergence of receptor theory of drug action (that specific drugs reacted with specific receptors in the body), helped to liken certain drugs to magic bullets.[23] This metaphor, which became increasingly used in the last decades of the twentieth century, had already been popularised to some extent in 1940 by the successful Hollywood movie, *Dr Ehrlich's Magic Bullet*, and by a short film by the US Public Health Service, *Magic Bullets*, one aspect of ongoing educational programmes against syphilis.[24]

In fact the military language of various public health promotion campaigns and studies is particularly potent in encouraging combative mindsets (e.g. the 'war on drugs', especially in the US). An interesting, almost subliminal, example of military mindsets is the appearance of uniformed Public Health Service officers in the 1997 movie version of *Miss Evers' Boys*, a story based on the US Public Health Service's 'Tuskegee Study' of the natural history of syphilis (1932–1973).[25] Central to the study, now recognised as infamous for its unethical/racial aspects, was the failure to give 'magic bullets' of penicillin to the untreated black men in the study, even after it became available to the general public in 1945–46.[26]

Movies and novels dealing with disease outbreaks have much potential to encourage notions of warfare by fostering public fears about disease. In the 1990s, widespread fascination with the Ebola virus is mirrored in *Outbreak* (1995) with its subplot of using the virus (called Motoba virus) for biological warfare. There is, too, persistent interest in possible outbreaks of plague and other decimating pandemics. Both *The Plague* (1993), a movie adaptation of Albert Camus' celebrated novel of the same title, and the period movie *Restoration* (1995) not only depict horrors of the disease, but are also a setting to real fears for many new problems from AIDS to SARS. It is easy to feel that science fiction plots are becoming true, or at least they are just around the corner – for instance, as in Peter Watts' dark novels, *Starfish* and *Maelstrom*, in which a non-DNA-using microbe is let loose from an undersea rift vent with the capacity to destroy all life.[27]

Given how the war on disease metaphor is so deeply embedded in society, we notice again the question whether it encourages vigorous treatment. Excessive prescribing of antibiotics is one obvious consideration. After all, it puzzles many why excessive prescribing persists among physicians amid frequent warnings of impending disaster from resistant organisms – warnings that have reached popular culture with article after article on superbugs or 'germs fight back'.[28]

Cancer merits special comment partly because the 'War on Cancer' was politically cemented in place in 1971 with President Richard Nixon's declaration of war on the disease with a new Cancer Act and new research funding. Even before then, however, vigorous interventionist treatment regimens were already well established. The correspondence of Rachel Carson (*see* Chapter 2) in the 1960s reveals her constant ordeal with various treatments as she was dying of breast cancer; this has led one commentator to observe that it 'becomes much easier to understand why the experience of cancer relies so heavily on military metaphors. The relentless succession of symptoms and side-effects that Carson experienced really was a bombardment. Over the last two years of her life, the pace seemed hardly to let up.'[29] It is plausible to suggest that a war on disease mindset helped to sustain invasive surgery of breast cancer (total mastectomy) rather than lumpectomy, which was generally resisted when promoted in the 1950s. In commenting on the radical operations current in the 1950s, the author of *The Breast Cancer Wars* considers that the language of war 'spoke to the surgical profession's ability to establish the criteria by which the successful treatment of cancer would be evaluated. As on the battlefield, courage and valor in the operating room would almost become ends in themselves';[30] this is not to say that surgeons did not rationalise the radical mastectomy operation developed by William Halstead on the basis of current theories of the spread of cancer accepted as the scientific underpinning of surgical intervention.[31]

Disease and stigma

Despite the widespread acceptance of war on disease metaphors, they have not escaped critical comment and were central to Susan Sontag's already mentioned attack on metaphors. In her mission to demystify disease, she wrote: 'the effect of the military imagery on thinking about sickness and health is far from inconsequential. It overmobilizes, it overdescribes, and it powerfully contributes to the excommunicating and stigmatizing of the ill.'[32] She adds, 'my point is that illness is *not* a metaphor, and that the most truthful way of regarding illness – and the healthiest way of being ill – is one most purified of, most resistant to, metaphoric thinking.'[33] In her concerns that military and other metaphors contribute to stigmatising sufferers from cancer and AIDS, Sontag opens questions such as whether a time-consuming patient who is 'not doing well' becomes a mere 'casualty' in the mind of his or her physician – perhaps dismissed as another 'case'.[34] In such an event, any consideration of alternative approaches to care may well be forestalled.

Unquestionably, metaphors can open doors to stigmatisation, if only because any person who departs from what is viewed as normal is commonly seen to be different. Popular culture has long stereotyped differences; persons with disabilities, for instance, have a traumatic history of being viewed as freaks, monsters with evil intent, obsessive avengers, asexual females, and more.[35] And sufferers from infectious diseases, e.g. leprosy, smallpox and syphilis, are set apart not only because of the fear they generate, but also because of resulting disfigurement and consequent labelling as being 'unclean'.[36] This has a long history; for instance, seventeenth-century poets and other writers on smallpox focused on 'beauty's enemy' as much as on mortality itself.[37] Further, the label 'unclean' extended to non-infectious skin ailments such as psoriasis, one of the conditions covered by the epithet *noli me tangere* until it was clearly distinguished from leprosy in the nineteenth century. Stigmas remain even in our so-called enlightened times. Kathleen Newroe is one of many who has written about psoriasis sufferers and the way it has affected them as individuals.[38] For a long time as a child, Newroe didn't notice that she was constantly scratching. However, when she was a teenager two commercials appeared. One was about how a guy would see a girl and think she looked great and then she'd itch her head and he'd be turned off.

> It didn't surprise me; this was what my mother had been telling me anyway, along with how I should wear lipstick and a girdle.
> But then there was the other one, about the 'heartbreak of psoriasis'.
> And that one did get to me because everyone laughed.
> It became a big joke, you know. You'd hear it everywhere. 'Oh, no! It's the heartbreak of psoriasis.' It was the sarcasm of the times.
> It offended me, though I wouldn't have known how to say so then. I mean, I had lived with psoriasis since I was eight and I wasn't walking around all day, everyday, with tears in my eyes. If I was the one who had it, and I could overlook it, I sure thought everyone else could, too.

New diseases are lightning rods for attracting stigmas, despite changing social values.[39] For instance, just as the widespread use of penicillin mitigated the stigma of syphilis from the 1960s onwards, AIDS, as a 'homosexual' disease (the way it was initially described), became the condition viewed as retribution for moral degradation. No amount of publicity about the spread of AIDS eliminated public fears of catching the disease in non-sexual ways.

> Friends venture toward my infected bed.
> They do not touch my blotched hand.
> My wife used to love me. Now,
> she enters in yellow gown and gloves.
> My mother fears my drool.[40]

As clinical decision makers, physicians must consider just how their own clinical objectiveness might be affected by disease stigmas. Physician–poet Dannie Abse opened a poem, 'Tuberculosis', with the lines:

> Not wishing to pronounce the taboo word
> I used to write, 'Acid-fast organisms'.[41]

Summary comments

Sontag's general attack on metaphors and stigma is not without foundation, but her particular arguments over cancer and tuberculosis, with a particular reliance on literary quotes, have been challenged.[42] For instance, one of her key points – a conspiracy of silence over cancer, a sense of shame – is questioned by evidence (from Canada) that much interchange of information between cancer sufferers took place at least prior to the Second World War.[43]

A much broader challenge to Sontag comes from the collective voices of autopathographies that suggest positive aspects to the war on disease mindset need to be considered; for instance, helping, even motivating, some patients to remain positive and to take responsibility for their care. Moreover, metaphors, especially those coined by patients themselves, can be part of coping, perhaps by finding meaning in or rationalising their condition. Caren Buffum, for instance, invoked a road rather than a candle:

> I think there is comfort in knowing that as I slip closer to the end of my life, it is not growing smaller like a candle being burned to the bottom. That in writing my story, even if the writing only selectively captures what my life has been about, it becomes less like that candle and more like a road – though traveled on, it continues to exist behind me.[44]

There are, too, reminders of views that extinguishing hope (say by a bluntly spoken diagnosis and prognosis), even in life-threatening situations, may not be in the best interest of the patient.[45]

Although possible downsides exist to military metaphors when patients feel that their 'battle' with a disease is being lost, it is difficult to conceive that metaphors in healthcare, so long embedded in our culture and medical language – evidenced by many byways of medical humanities, for example political prints – will ever be eliminated.[46] Nevertheless, Sontag prompts our thinking not only on the role of metaphor, but also stereotyping illness and people. Thus she adds to the jolts that many a visual artist can give to the way we stereotype people. Alice Neel's nude self-portrait when aged eighty, for example is difficult to dismiss. As has been said, 'many viewers are caught off guard by Neel's reinterpretation of the gazed upon nude. Seated in a chair, and without apparent concern for sagging breasts and folds of skin on chin, abdomen and thighs, the subject looks directly at the viewer through large glasses as an engaged participant in what has been called the 'duality of being, the self as observer and observed'.[47]

Such challenges should provoke practitioners to listen more intently to the use of metaphors and stereotypes in medical and everyday language, to recognise the need to understand and evaluate them, and to ask whether they shape their own clinical decision making.

Endnotes

1 Baldwin F (1945) *Medical Center*. Blakiston, Philadelphia (reprint of 1940), p. 4.
2 Peabody FW (1930) *Doctor and Patient*. The Macmillan Company, New York, pp. 22–3. Even one homeopathic physician expressed (1912) concerns over the seductiveness of diagnosis at the expense of attention of the minutiae of homeopathic treatments: Scwartz WH (1912) Diagnosis vs. the homoeopathic prescription. *The Homoeopathician*. **1** (1): 35–7.
3 To give one example, the website of University Physicians at Texas Tech Medical Center indicates that internists are sometimes referred to as diagnosticians: www.ama.ttuhsc.edu/UniversityPhysicians/im/ (accessed July 2004).
4 Davies R (1994) *The Cunning Man*. McClelland and Stewart, Toronto.
5 Quoted in Introduction by Elliott C and Lantos J (eds) (1999) *The Last Physician: Walker Percy & the moral life of medicine*. Duke University Press, Durham, p. 4 (emphasis added). That Percy maintained a doctor's mindset in illuminating the vicissitudes of human connectedness: Coles R (1999) Dr Percy's hold on medicine. Ibid., pp. 9–13. Recent review, Montogomery GJP (2004) Diagnosing dis-ease: Dr Walker Percy and the pathology of modern malaise. In: Whitelaw WA (ed) *Proceedings of the 13th Annual History of Medicine Days*. Faculty of Medicine, University of Calgary, Calgary, pp. 226–32.
6 Quoted in Coles (1999) Dr Percy's hold on medicine, p. 13.

7   For significance of concept of specificity, Crellin JK (2004) *A Social History of Medicines in the Twentieth Century. To Be Taken Three Times a Day.* Haworth Press, New York, especially pp. 165–6. The issue of the pharmaceutical industry's influence on diagnosis has attracted much attention in recent years. For instance, around the time of writing, Moyhihan R (2003) drew attention to certain issues in: The making of a disease: female sexual dysfunction. *British Medical Journal.* **326**: 45–7.

8   It should perhaps be added that, despite the popular appeal of complementary and alternative medicine, Hollywood has not been overly kind to the growth of complementary alternative medicine, often suggesting it is mere quackery. Cf. the movies *H.E.A.L.T.H.* (1979) and *The Road to Wellville* (1994).

9   *Dr AW Chase's Calendar Almanac 1936.* Dr AW Chase Medicine Co., Toronto, p. 35.

10 Baldwin (1945) *Medical Center*, pp. 17–18.

11 The increasingly complex world of multicultural societies constantly raises communication problems. Of many books to capture this, see O'Connor BB (1995) *Healing Traditions: alternative medicine and the health professions.* University of Pennsylvania Press, Philadelphia.

12 Querry R (1998) *Bad Medicine.* Bantam Books, New York.

13 For background to the above statements, Crellin (2004) *A Social History of Medicines in the Twentieth Century.* As for certain physicians' reputations for their medicines, these have not always depended entirely on pharmacological efficacy. Considerations of palatability were important; many medicines, at least up to around the 1940s, were 'known' for high alcohol content.

14 Sontag S (1978) *Illness as Metaphor* has been reprinted with a new essay as *Illness as Metaphor and Aids and its Metaphors.* Doubleday, New York, 1990.

15 Quote from Irving Wilson Voorhees. In: Huth EJ and Murray TJ (eds) (2000) *Medicine in Quotations: views of health and disease through the ages.* American College of Physicians, Philadelphia, p. 157.

16 Quote from Budd Schulberg. In: Strauss MB (ed) (1968) *Familiar Medical Quotations.* Little, Brown and Company, Boston, p. 385.

17 Personal communication, Caroline Blackman.

18 Virshup B (1985) *How to Cope with Your Doctor.* Praxis Press, Woodland Hills, pp. 39–40, for one commentator who divides physicians into two categories.

19 Warner JH (1977–1978) 'The nature-trusting Heresy': American physicians and the concept of the healing power of nature in the 1850s and 1860s. *Perspectives in American History.* **11**: 291–324.

20 It must be stressed that, as noted, some physicians are watchers. Moreover, public concerns with side-effects of medications mean that more caution is being exercised with prescription products.

21 Nuland SB (1997) *The Wisdom of the Body.* Knopf, New York, p. 278.

22 Notions of war on disease seemingly extend back as far as ancient Greece as evidenced in Thucydides' account of the Athenian plague in his *History of the Peloponnesian War* (trans by CF Smith) (1935) Harvard University Press, Cambridge.

23 For some context, Parascandola J and Jasensky R (1974) Origins of the receptor theory of drug action. *Bulletin of the History of Medicine.* **48**: 199–220. It should be added that a big impetus to the idea of the magic bullet came with the introduction of sulphonamides. It is appropriate to add that social factors within science can be relevant to the development of a concept (such as 'magic bullet') as made clear in an essay on Paul Fildes (1882–1971), who argued that chemicals with a structure similar to an essential metabolite of a microorganism could delude an organism into thinking that the drug is an essential metabolite. See Kohler RE (1985) Bacterial physiology: the medical context. *Bulletin of the History of Medicine.* **59**: 54–74.

24 For background and use of the magic bullet metaphor, Lederer S and Parascandola J (1998) Screening syphilis: *Dr Ehrlich's Magic Bullet* meets the public health service. *Journal of the History of Medicine.* **53**: 345–70.

25 The movie is based on the play of the same title by David Feldshuh, who is both a physician and artistic director of the Cornell Center for Theatre Arts; he has a special interest in the use of the theatre to explore important social issues. www.arts.cornell.edu/theatrearts/Feldshuh.html (accessed February 2002).

26 E.g. Reverby S (2000) *Tuskegee's Truths: rethinking the Tuskegee Syphilis Study*. University of North Carolina Press, Chapel Hill.

27 *Starfish*. Tor, New York, 1999; *Maelstrom*. Tor, New York, 2001.

28 E.g. recently Shnayerson M and Plotkin MJ (2002) *The Killers Within: the deadly rise of drug-resistant bacteria*. Little, Brown and Company, Boston.

29 Leopold E (1999) *A Darker Ribbon: breast cancer, women and their doctors in the twentieth century*. Beacon Press, Boston, p. 149.

30 Lerner BH (2001) *The Breast Cancer Wars: hope, fear and the pursuit of a cure in twentieth-century America*. Oxford University Press, Oxford, p. 69. Also, Lerner BH, Fighting the 'War' on Breast Cancer: how a metaphor has shaped the debate on early detection and treatment: www.cpmcnet.Columbia.edu/news/journal/archives/jour_v19no1/breast.html (accessed February 2003).

31 See, for example, Saunders-Goebel P (1991) Crisis and controversy: historical patterns in breast surgery. *Canadian Bulletin Medical History*. **8**: 77–90. At issue is whether the disease is primarily local and spreading out or is basically a systemic disease.

32 Quoted in Semmler IA (1998) Ebola goes pop: the filovirus from literature into film. *Literature and Medicine*. **17**: 149–74. From Sontag (1990) *Illness as Metaphor and AIDS and its Metaphors*, p. 182. It should be noted that Sontag's critique, at least aspects of it, have not gone unchallenged, for instance Clow B (2001) Who's afraid of Susan Sontag? Or, the myths and metaphors of cancer reconsidered.' *Social History of Medicine*. **14**: 293–312.

33 Sontag (1990) *Illness as Metaphor and AIDS and its Metaphors*, p. 3.

34 Ibid., p. 99. Sontag saw the language of 'case', particularly with cancer, as a stigma, a diminution of the self, inhibiting people from seeking treatment early. She was equally damming of the negative associations with AIDS, such as seeing it as plague-like, a moral judgement on society (p. 148). It seems appropriate to add that the war on disease offers little incentive to consider other theoretical approaches, such as to view disease in the individual and in society within the context of evolution. The authors of, for instance, *Evolution and Healing* (1995) make clear that they are not urging an alternative to modern medical practice, but 'rather an additional perspective from a well-established body of scientific knowledge [about adaptation and historical causation] that has been largely neglected by the medical profession.' (Nesse RM and Williams GW (1995) *Evolution and Healing*. Weidenfield and Nicolson, London, p. xi.)

35 Cf. Norden MF (1994) *The Cinema of Isolation: a history of physical disability in the movies*. Rutgers University Press, New Brunswick, pp. 314–23.

36 Syphilis, it should be remembered, can produce skin lesions, though stigma also comes from implications of loose morals and the decay of the social order.

37 The title of a poem by Thomas Shipman (1632–1680): Beauty's enemy: upon the death of M Princess of Orange, by the smallpox. In *Carolina: Or Loyal Poems*. (1683) Facsimile Reproduction Scholars' Facsimiles and Reprints, 1980. pp. 78–9. I am grateful to Iona Bulgin for this reference.

38 Newroe K (1992) Psoriasis. In: Walker SB and Roffman RD *Life on the Line: selections on words and healing*. Negative Capability Press, Mobile, pp. 280–1. See also Meulenberg F (1997) The hidden delight of psoriasis. *British Medical Journal*. **315**: 1709–11.

39 Changing social attitudes are well demonstrated in the social attitudes that emerged in the last years of the twentieth century, namely a commonplace stigmatisation of smokers, an aspect of the tendency to blame people for their ill health.

40 Verse from 'AIDS' by Elspeth Cameron Ritchie in Walker SB and Roffman RD (eds) (1992) *Life on the Line: selections on words and healing*. Negative Capability Press, Mobile, p. 211.

41 Quoted in Walker and Roffman (1992) *Life on the Line*, p. 277.

42 It is instructive to note that many of Sontag's references to metaphors come from literary texts. She is, for example, critical of the Romantic cult associated with tuberculosis in the nineteenth century – 'as a sign of superior nature, as a becoming frailty.' (*Illness as Metaphor and AIDS and its Metaphors*. p. 34.) Yet Sontag herself points out that this was not universal. Death from tuberculosis could be a redemptive death for the fallen, like the prostitute Fantine in *Les Misérables*, or a sacrificial death for the virtuous, like the heroine of Selma Lagerlöf's *The Phantom Chariot*, but it could also be associated with the stigma of poverty (ibid., pp. 41–2.)

43 Clow (2001) Who's afraid of Susan Sontag? Or the myths and metaphors of cancer reconsidered.

44 Quoted from 'Stress, personality and metaphors of illness', Mayer M (1998) *Advanced Breast Cancer: a guide to living with metastatic disease.* O'Reilly & Associates, Inc. through www.patientcenters.com/breastcancer/news/stress_metaphors.html (accessed July 2004). For other comments on roles of metaphors embedded in society: Weinstein A (2003) Afterword: infection as metaphor. *Literature and Medicine.* **22**: 102–15.

45 The role of hope occasions a great deal of debate. Cf. Kodish E and Post SG (1995) Oncology and hope. *Journal of Clinical Oncology.* **13**: 1817–22. Also of interest, comments on the tyranny of positive thinking in Holland JC and Lewis S (2000) *Living with Hope, Coping with Uncertainty.* HarperCollins, New York, pp. 13–25.

46 One byway of medical humanities, which also points up the cultural presence of analogies between medicine and everyday life in an entertaining way, is political prints. Although perhaps commenting little on disease, they often point up the power, if not the abuse of power, of the physician as they satirically invoke a political event, a new piece of legislation, or an unpopular politician, etc. Political prints, albeit with their golden age in eighteenth- and nineteenth-century Britain, and in the US around the time of the civil war, still have an impact, although only a relative few are as biting as their predecessors.

   Such prints with medical themes, in viewing the political body as suffering from all manner of ailments, also serve to highlight medical practices of the time and the 'fight' against disease. A tug of war, if not a battle, is often seen between a physician (with his bitter pills, enemas and lancets for bleeding) and a patient (representing the opposition, the unpopular policy, the enemy, etc). One fairly common scene in early prints, French ones in particular, is a physician brandishing an enema syringe as if it is a weapon. Less evocative is Art Stradler's 1982 political postcard (author's collection) that shows President Ronald Reagan as a surgeon pushing a needle (some might see this as a weapon) into the grossly expanded abdomen of a woman. The caption, 'Doc Reagan says: "Abolish Waist and Reduce Inflation"', is an obvious reminder of late twentieth-century preoccupation with obesity, or, to use another war metaphor, the battle of the bulge. Moreover, the cartoon may be seen to question the power of the physician and the politician.

47 Discussed in Nixon LL and Roscoe LA (2002) Anticipating deep autumn: a widening lens. *Medical Humanities Edition of the Journal of Medical Ethics.* **28**: 82–7.

CHAPTER 10

Caged, controlled, classified

In continuing to look at attitudes, metaphors and stereotypes that can have an impact on clinical decisions, this chapter focuses particular attention on whether patients feel caged, trapped or classified. Although the feelings are especially conspicuous among neurology and psychiatry patients, they can be found among a wide range of patients – for some it is any departure from the often difficult-to-define 'normal'.[1] Moreover, the chapter also looks at gender stereotyping, which is both an obvious and subtle form of classification that affects countless patients. Clearly, these are matters for all practitioners to consider, even if they do not necessarily have obvious medical consequences such as a direct impact on medication decisions. Yet clinical decisions can be affected in subtle ways insofar as understanding patients' feelings can play a role in empathising with patients and appreciating their needs. In comments on empathy in Chapter 4, it was said that empathy can be cultivated through 'informed imagination'. Exploring caging/stereotyping is an important aspect of this.

The feeling of 'being caged' by disease has been expressed in many ways – of being a 'caged animal', a 'caged butterfly', of being trapped in a bell-jar.[2] Others can feel trapped by being labelled or stereotyped. Although metaphors likening disease to being caged or trapped are much less evident than war on disease metaphors, caged feelings can be felt by patients suffering from almost any condition. Albert Camus, too, makes clear in his now classic novel, *The Plague* (1947), that a person can feel controlled or imprisoned by a disease in many ways.[3] The frailty of old age is just one instance:

> Caged! he thought with a fury that was no good at all for his heart. Caged with a senile smiling keeper. At times he had to restrain himself from punching out the screen with his bare fists and catapulting his body over the sill for the sheer pleasure of unimpeded movement. It was a seductive ending: to lie broken-backed in the smashed lilacs, mouth full of warm June mud, taking a host of living things with him, vengeful as Samson.
> How delightfully embarrassing and humiliating it would be for Jason.[4]

Patients can signal a sense of being caged in various ways. Always thought-provoking are the postcards mailed by hospital patients who have marked the window of their hospital room or ward with an X. Gazing at the windows of a hospital, especially if a close friend or relative is inside, can be as emotional for a visitor as it is for a patient who longs to be on the outside. James Dickey's poem 'The Hospital Window' is about a son, who, after visiting a dying father, scans tiers of hospital windows knowing that his father lies behind one of them. The son, however, is able to feel a connection, and hence acquire some sense of healing.[5]

Caged by neurological disease

Feelings of being caged are particularly prevalent among those suffering from neurological and psychiatric conditions as has been underscored by various narratives published in recent years. Although issues are fairly clear in the fascinating and well-known examples considered next, they continually challenge practitioners to understand the 'whole' person, and perhaps to reconsider any initial, perhaps superficial, impressions they have of a patient.

Oliver Sacks, a neurologist, has written a great deal on people who must feel caged. Only a few commentators consider he 'exploits' patients, perhaps as freaks, for his narratives are generally seen as revealing persons with sensitivities, feelings, insights and special abilities to cope with their disabilities.[6] Especially well known among Sacks' writings is *Awakenings* (1973), in part because of the successful movie version.[7] The book comprises 'third person' histories (that is, written by Sacks who calls them 'person', not 'case' histories) of patients suffering from the sequelae of encephalitis lethargica. This, also known as von Economo disease, is assumed to be a viral disease that was epidemic following World War I.[8] Long-term symptoms resemble a severe form of Parkinson's disease with total rigidity, or mummification to use Sacks' term. After levodopa (L-dopa) became accepted treatment for Parkinson's disease in 1967, Sacks tried it (in 1969) on his patients with dramatic results.

A particularly insightful person history centres on Leonard L, largely because, as Sacks indicated, Leonard combined 'the profoundest disease with the acutest investigative intelligence.'[9] Leonard had the ability to express vividly how he felt being 'Caged. Deprived. Like Rilke's Panther', 'of being trapped inside myself', of being 'castrated by my illness, and relieved from all the longings other people have.'[10] Sacks first provides a detailed picture of Leonard before treatment when he could only answer questions by painfully tapping out answers on a letter board. His answers were often telegraphic and sometimes cryptic. He expressed feelings of violence and power, which were 'locked up' inside him. 'I have no exit,' he would tap out. 'I am trapped in myself. This stupid body is a prison with windows but no doors.'[11]

The course of Leonard's condition – his 'sudden conversion' and the sequelae – after L-dopa was started in March 1969 is the core of Leonard's story, which has much to say about hopes and uncertainties brought about by modern drugs. Early on, the rigidity diminished in Leonard's limbs, he felt energy and power, was able to write and type once again, to rise from his chair, to walk with some assistance, and to speak in a loud and clear voice. Everything filled Leonard with delight as if awakened from a nightmare. He became intoxicated with the sense of beauty around him. His readings of the classics such as Dante's *Paradismo* took on new meanings. 'I feel saved,' he would say, 'resurrected, re-born. I feel a sense of health amounting to Grace ... I feel like a man in love.'[12]

The unhappy part of the story is that the positive effects of L-dopa did not persist. In evocative language, Sacks describes how Leonard's sense of harmony and ease and effortless control was replaced by a sense of too muchness, of force and pressure, and a pulling apart. Contrasting sharply to the pre-L-Dopa frozen state, manic behaviour took over. As Leonard's demeanour worsened, reading became difficult because of uncontrollable hurry and repetitive behaviour. Once he had started he would read faster and faster without regard for the sense or syntax, and, unable to stop, he would have to shut the book with a snap after each sentence or paragraph in order to digest its sense. He also developed sudden impulsions and tics of the eyes, grimaces, cluckings and lightning-quick scratchings. Leonard's final effort at control was to write his autobiography, which came to 50 000 words in length. Unfortunately, when finished, Leonard's state passed beyond all bounds of control.

Sacks closes his narrative with Leonard's words – a comment on one of the most humbling of therapeutic experiments: 'It is finally – *sad*, and that's all there is to it. I'm best left alone – no more drugs. I've learned a great deal in the last three years. I've broken through barriers which I had all my life. And now, I'll stay myself, and you can keep your L-Dopa.'[13] Leonard was reasserting a view he had expressed before he took L-dopa: 'My disease and deformity are part of the world. They are beautiful in a way like a dwarf or a toad. It's my destiny to be a sort of grotesque.'[14] *Awakenings*, like much of Sacks writings, undoubtedly challenge healthcare practitioners to understand how patients come to terms with, and sometimes find comfort within, their sick role.

Another startling case of 'being caged' is recorded in an autobiography by a sufferer of locked-in syndrome. This condition results from damage to the brain stem such as by a stroke; a patient is paralysed in all four extremities but retains consciousness. Jean-Dominique Bauby was so stricken in 1995 when aged 43. He was left with one movement – the ability to blink his left eyelid with which he was able to acknowledge letters of the alphabet read out to him. He was thus able to 'dictate' what he called his 'bedridden travel notes'.[15] He described his condition with such metaphors as 'something like a giant invisible diving-bell [that] holds my whole body prisoner,' and a mind that takes 'flight like a butterfly'.[16] The travel notes, extraordinarily entertaining and insightful despite the pathos of Bauby's situation, are a mix of sharp memories and acute observations on surroundings, on visitors, and on an array of care-givers. Some of the latter were thoughtful and humane, while others treated Bauby like a vegetable.

While he gave accolades to his speech therapist ('an angel'), his harsh judgement about an ophthalmologist is as strong a patient's challenge to physicians as can be found anywhere. He describes how on a late January morning the hospital ophthalmologist was leaning over him and sewing his right eyelid shut with a 'needle and thread, just as if he were darning a sock'. Bauby describes how 'irrational terror swept over me. What if this man got carried away and sewed up my left eye as well, my only link to the outside world, the only window to my cell, the one tiny opening of my cocoon?' Although this did not happen, the physician, on leaving, barked in the ...

> tones of a prosecutor demanding a maximum sentence for a repeat offender ... 'Six months!' I fired off a series of questioning signals with my working eye, but this man – who spent his days looking into other people's pupils – was apparently unable to interpret a simple look. He was the very model of the couldn't care less doctor, arrogant, brusque, sarcastic, the kind who summons his patients for 8.00 a.m., arrives at 9.00, and departs at 9.05 after giving each one forty-five seconds of his precious time.

Bauby adds that, already disinclined to chat with normal patients, the physician turned thoroughly evasive in dealing with 'ghosts of my ilk'. After discovering that the closing of his eye was because the eyelid no longer fulfilled its protective function and thus he risked an ulcerated cornea, Bauby went on to muse. Did the hospital employ such an ungracious character deliberately to serve as a focal point for the veiled mistrust the medical profession always arouses in long-term patients? 'A kind of scapegoat, in other words.'[17] Bauby also harshly judged lay people who stereotyped his condition as being nothing more than a 'vegetable'. His quip that he would 'have to rely on myself if I wanted to prove that my IQ was still higher than a turnip' revealed an indomitable spirit unlikely to be found in those who dismissed him.[18]

A third neurological example of being caged became especially well known through the movie version of the story of John Merrick (1862–1890), the 'Elephant Man'. Merrick, grossly deformed from an extreme case of neurofibromatosis (tumours along the myelin sheaths of nerves), was 'discovered' by Frederick Treves, a London surgeon, who found a home for Merrick in the London Hospital.

Writing in 1923 – a time when those with disabilities were commonly viewed as freaks and, like Merrick, still destined to become fairground exhibits – Treves noted that Merrick had become as secluded from the world as the 'Man with the Iron Mask'.[19] Although initially believing Merrick to be an 'imbecile from birth', Treves came to know him as 'highly intelligent' with an 'acute sensibility'. Treves, too, recognised that Merrick's romantic imagination underscored the 'overwhelming tragedy of his life'.

Treves describes his treatment – a form of psychotherapy to rid Merrick's mind of his fears – as helping Merrick to become accustomed to *human* beings. 'He got to know most of the people about the place, to be accustomed to their comings and goings, and to realise that they took no more than a friendly notice of him.' Merrick also became well acquainted with women in Treves' own social circle. Recovering some of his imagination led to Merrick's transformation in spirit, even in his secluded quarters at the hospital. He pushed aside the thought of wishing to live in a 'blind asylum or to a lighthouse'. 'He had read about blind asylums in the newspapers and was attracted by the thought of being among people who could not see.' The lighthouse had another charm. It meant seclusion from the curious. There at least no one could open a door and peep in at him. There he would forget that he had once been the Elephant Man.

Of special interest in terms of people finding meanings or explanations for their condition (*see* healing, Chapter 4) is Merrick's story that his mother had been frightened shortly before his birth when she had been knocked down by an elephant in a circus.[20] Analogous folklore on the negative outcomes of frights during pregnancy, albeit faded, may still be an issue today.

Readers, whether health professionals or not, will consider the above three examples far removed from everyday issues facing physicians. Yet there is one common feature to consider, namely the presence of the onlooker. The sense of being caged invariably depends on the presence of voyeurs – always an issue, but especially obvious with regard to mental health as considered next. The message, for practitioners and lay people alike, is to consider how to avoid being perceived as a voyeur.

Trapped by voyeurism and the stigma of society

> There was a wall of silence from the medical establishment, I got no help from doctors. They observed me like a caged animal, watching how my brain worked by making me play Scrabble. (A sufferer from schizophrenia)[21]

One picture to reappear continually in medical books, at least those devoted to history, is a scene from *The Rake's Progress* (1735) by William Hogarth. It depicts two ladies of fashion viewing the mentally ill in a ward at London's Bethlem Hospital; they are peering into a cell of a naked man wearing only a crown while other inmates 'perform' in various ways. Historians have noted how it was a pastime for members of the public to visit Bethlem. 'It was deliberately putting the Other on show, a blatant form of voyeurism.'[22] Hogarth's picture can prompt the question whether, today, voyeurism exacerbates the stigma felt by those who suffer from what has been called the most solitary of afflictions.[23]

Although Bethlem Hospital's exploitation of the mentally ill (visitors were expected to make a donation) has gone, as have chains and shackles for the mentally ill (albeit replaced by what some see as 'chemical restraints'), movies have long offered a similar, if second-hand, brand of voyeurism – and without financial donation to the care of the ill. Negative movie images began in the early days of silent movies with, for example, *The Escaped Lunatic* (1904), *Maniac Chase* (1904) and *Dr Dippy's Sanitarium* (1906). Of the variety of images and stereotypes, the commonplace image of hospitalised ('incarcerated') mentally ill patients with excessively bizarre behaviours is most conspicuous. Recent comedy examples – often with affinities to Hogarth's scene in *The Rake's Progress* – are found in *The Dream Team* (1989) and *Crazy People* (1990). Contrasting horrendous images appear in what were intended, in part, as exposés of mental institutions: *The Snake Pit* (1948), *Chattahooche* (1989) and *Beautiful Dreamers* (1996). In *The Snake Pit*, one of the first films to reveal the many inadequacies of US state mental institutions, the principal character, Virginia Cunningham, comments on the similarities between hospitalised patients on the wards and caged animals in the zoo. Sometimes images are shaped to reflect specific worries of the time; for instance, homicidal maniacs such as in *Psycho II* (1983) and *Psycho III* (1986) seemingly carry a message that such individuals, after being 'cured,' revert back to their homicidal ways.[24]

Even if the precise impact of unsympathetic movie images of mental illness cannot be measured, it is hard to believe that they do not contribute to stigmatisation of mental illness. Moreover, this impacts on families of mentally handicapped persons, who may feel, too, that they are on display, trapped or caged. Novels such as Kaye Gibbons' *Sights Unseen* (1995), which tells of a girl growing up in North Carolina with a manic depressive mother, are just as telling as many an academic writing in asking physicians for family care.[25]

One striking aspect of Hollywood's depictions of mental illness, especially when psychiatry is very much part of the main plot, is that the psychiatrist may be shown to be as much in need of help as the patient.[26] Although we are presently considering the role of voyeur in contributing to the stigma of mentally ill patients, lay attitudes can also be coloured by perceptions of psychiatry in general – in seeing it as a world apart.

One of the most striking features of the recent history of medicine is the fall from grace of psychiatrists from their golden Hollywood period – very much part of the negative imagery of physicians discussed in Chapter 2. This is to be seen in the context of various factors that have had public impact, of which movies are just one. Another has been the 'anti-psychiatry movement', especially prominent in the 1960s.[27] Spearheading the movement were critics from within psychiatry such as Thomas Szasz and RD Laing; they questioned the existence of mental disease and argued that persons with deviant views might well be the more enlightened members of society because they rejected society's constricting conventions.[28] More recently, widespread public concerns over psychiatry have been compounded by ongoing controversies over, for example, the way various psychiatric disorders are diagnosed, the countless stories about over-medication (e.g. by Valium and Prozac), and the suspicions over psychoanalysis, viewed by many as without adequate empirical and theoretical foundations.[29]

It has been said that negative screen images of psychiatry adversely affect patients by causing them to over-idealise or to distrust their psychiatrists. In a detailed discussion, Krin and Glen Gabbard (1999) point out that the answer to the question whether screen portrayals of psychiatrists are accurate is 'yes' and 'no'. There really are psychiatrists, they say, who are sadistic and punitive towards their patients; psychoanalysts who act on their erotic feelings towards their own patients; and 'probably even instances of psychiatrists who have murdered their own patients.'[30] Moreover, 'psychiatric patients come to the consulting room with expectations of how a psychiatrist should behave based on what they see in movies.' Many feel, like the Gabbards, that 'media images insidiously work their way into the collective unconscious of society and influence the way we all regard the world around us.'[31]

Gender and health: what to make of stereotypes?

Of all the socio-cultural issues than can impinge on clinical decision making, gender stereotyping – bound closely with a sense of being classified if not caged or otherwise controlled – is high on any list. Physicians often fail to recognise the complex boundaries that society places around gender and sexuality in general, and that these make all practitioners especially vulnerable to overstepping the boundaries. In fact, society in recent years, as noted in Chapter 2, has increased its scrutiny of the sanctions it gives physicians that allow physical examinations and treatment.

Inappropriate boundary-crossing raises the question whether physicians sometimes slide into unprofessional situations because of their general discomfort with sexuality – their own, their patients, or both – and their inexperience with transference and counter-transference of emotional feelings between themselves and patients.[32] In fact, public voices question whether physicians, in general, have sufficient understanding of societal/cultural attitudes towards gender and sexuality, as distinct from detailed knowledge of the anatomy and physiology of sexual organs and functions. Certainly, criticisms exist over limited formal education (or even informal teaching) on sexuality in most medical schools. Even when 'women's health' is a designated part of a curriculum, there is rarely a learning environment that enables students to become familiar with cultural factors shaping human sexuality (their own included), ignorance of which increases their chances of stereotyping patients. Few opportunities exist to explore many voices in the humanities that prompt introspection into one's own sexual values and behaviour; the voices range, for instance, from the physician in Miles Kunderer's acclaimed *Everyday Lightness of Being* to the movie *Boxing Helena* (1993) with its portrayal of a surgeon's grotesque sexual fantasy. Of course, such voices need to be placed within the context of the gender of the viewer and of the culture of society in general. Physicians, male and female, have to consider their attitudes to patients of the same and opposite sex. Here we illustrate some issues from relatively well-studied topics in order to encourage some introspection.

During the last half of the twentieth century, academia and popular culture pounced on gender, sexuality and health and gave it the pedigree of being a 'discipline' to be studied. Historians have contributed much to the new interest by revealing a variety of past episodes that raise questions about gender bias and male physician power. The 'modern' story of the stereotyping of women is commonly set in the context of a legacy of nineteenth-century views, albeit with earlier roots (cf. Box 10.1).

Box 10.1   Stereotyping sick women in the seventeenth century

Although this chapter is not concerned with the history of the concept of weakness in women, noticed here is Laurinda Dixon's study of numerous seventeenth-century Dutch genre paintings dealing with the themes of the lovesick maiden and a doctor's visit to an ailing woman who is 'usually young, pretty and well-dressed – [and] propped up in a chair or languishing in bed.' In some paintings, the woman has swooned and lies senseless.

Dixon argues that 'the image of the fragile, passive, housebound woman has always been a reflection more of male wish fulfillment than of female reality.' In supporting her overall theme, she offers fascinating interpretation about how medical knowledge of a period offers specific insights into the pictures. For instance, two paintings by Jan Steen depict a young man in the sickroom holding up a dead herring in the right hand and a bunch of onions in the other. Traditionally these foods have been seen as symbols, the herring representing folly, unchastity and licentiousness and the onion symbols of male testes and penis, both suggesting that the young girl is pregnant. On the other hand, Dixon, in considering a common diagnosis at the time (hysteria due to uterine problems that could affect all parts of the body) and contemporary knowledge of Galenic humours and the properties of food, suggests the two items can be interpreted in other ways: to bring on the menses, to deal with anorexia, or to satisfy a food craving. (Dixon LS (1995) *Perilous Chastity in Pre-Enlightenment Art and Medicine*. Cornell University Press, Ithaca, quotes pp. 1–3, 86–91.)

Particular attention is given to the way women were considered to be inherently weaker than men. Perceived tendencies to nervousness and to a general weakness – conditions linked to the 'special nature' of their reproductive organs – had pervasive effects on healthcare.[33] Many examples, straddling the eighteen and early nineteen hundreds, suggest that the cultural acceptance of the inherent weakness of women supported physicians who made it part of their diagnoses. One example is the marketing of countless patent or over-the-counter medicines that were directed specifically to the various ills of women. One North American manufacturer's promotional literature (1862) included the widely held view that a fundamental issue was the fine and complicated 'system of the *female*', more complex than that of men because of its double function of 'sustaining her own life, and giving life to her species'. Thus 'the wisdom of God', which gave a woman the peculiar 'sanguinous monthly discharge from the organs of generation' during child-bearing years, meant, as was argued, that she was subjected to far more frequent medical problems than a man. The writer adds that *debility* and *irregularities* are so inter-woven together that what causes one must necessarily affect the other.[34] Many over-the-counter medicines like 'Dr Pierce's Favorite Prescription' (a strong competitor for many decades to the more widely known Lydia Pinkham's Veg-etable Tonic) stressed the value of tonic effects on female nerves: 'it quiets nervous irritation, it strengthens the enfeebled nervous system, restoring it to healthful vigor. In an irritable condition of the nervous system, it is unsurpassed as a remedy. It is also a general tonic of great excellence. It is sold by all druggists.'[35]

The cultural presence of the concept of the inherent weakness of women does not mean that the specific influence of physician authority was unimportant. One illustration of this is the work of Philadelphia physician Silas Weir Mitchell (1829–1914). He became well known not only as a novelist, but also for his 'rest cure' treatment for women suffering from neurasthenia and like conditions. The 'cure' comprised a strict regimen of almost total bed rest (for six weeks or more), limited time for reading, complete nursing care, simple diet and no medications; the only stimulation was massage and electricity. Although very widely used, with many imitations, it did not go unchallenged.

One challenge to Mitchell was from author Charlotte Perkins Gilman, who 'suffered' through the rest cure and was one of a number of Victorian women whose invalidism, associated in particular with nervousness and weakness, became known well beyond local circles.[36] Her short story *The Yellow Wallpaper*, published 1892, clearly based on her own experiences, questioned the effectiveness, at least for her situation. Unfortunately her post-partum depression deepened during the rest cure. In particular, her dislike of the unclean, yellow-patterned wallpaper in the room where she was confined became such an obsession that, in the end, she attacked it and stripped it off. Her writing makes clear that she was in disagreement with physicians, one of whom was her husband, over treatment and believed that finding new ways to stimulate the mind had to be part of recovery. In recent decades the story has had a new life as it became a significant text in many women's studies classes that fostered women's rights.

The above comments focus on belief in the inherent weakness of women, but other factors have been identified by historians as contributing to cultural stereo-typing. Ludmilla Jordanova's stimulating book, *Sexual Visions: images of gender in science and medicine between the eighteenth and twentieth centuries* (1989), concluded that women and their secrets, like nature, 'have a profoundly ambiguous status, being both desired and feared' by men.[37] It has, too, been suggested, with regard to fear, that women were targeted viewers of numerous public health films produced between the late 1930s and the middle 1950s to promote public knowledge about tuberculosis. Significantly, the women were not 'the privileged objects of medical concern but ... representative bearers of contagious and insidiously hidden infection.'[38] Novels about colonial Africa also raise negative connotations insofar as they reflect that 'the association of Black women and disease' was commonplace.[39] Movies depicting psychiatrists raise additional ambivalent images. One stereotype, persisting in movies since the 1940s, is that women practitioners are more likely than male practitioners to be 'cured' of their own ills as a result of the physician–patient relationship. Perhaps, a 'message' from this is that women cannot have it all. Even when a woman psychotherapist successfully treats a patient, she is often presented as an unfulfilled spinster or divorcée.[40]

Much of the recent historical writing on female gender closes with comments on continuing issues in modern times, though this sometimes reflects feminist ideology rather than careful interpretation of the historical data. Yet continuums with the past clearly exist. Jordanova, in challenging opinions that gender biases are no longer visualised in our 'current, rationalistic environment', states that 'nothing, in my view, could be further from the truth ... The sexual ambiguity, the fantasies, the shades of violence, the collective investment in the nature of femininity still exist.'[41] Perhaps, too, there remain male attitudes explicit and implicit in the many sagas of 'pioneer' women entering medicine.[42] Another writer, Laurinda Dixon, sees a continuum subsequent to the depictions of women's weakness or frailty by seventeenth-century Dutch artists (*see* Box 10.1). In drawing attention to a 1966 advertisement depicting a mother/housewife who needs a tranquilliser to deal with the 'pressures [that] last all day,'[43] Dixon concludes:

> The study of depictions of women and illness suggests that no subject is more determined by contemporary cultural and social factors. Throughout history men have created images of women as reflections of male interests, anxieties and longings. They have invoked science in general and medicine in particular to justify the mandates of sex and class imposed on women by the powerful social order. Physicians have seen themselves as both moral and medical guardians of the 'weaker' sex, responding to an ancient and persistent belief in the inherent instability of women.

Many people, in accepting such sentiments, see them as continuing in the twenty-first century not only in advertising, but also in a range of unconscious attitudes expressed in, for instance, obstetricians' colloquialisms like 'lazy uterus' or 'incompetent cervix' or in sceptical attitudes toward chronic fatigue syndrome, a condition that particularly affects women. Concerns about biases also exist over medicalisation of childbirth, and in other aspects of women's health.[44] For instance, women feel that often their complaints are dismissed as psychological or 'all in the mind'. Some of this lies behind the statement that some 70 per cent of women who contact the Endometriosis Association have been told at least once that their symptoms are psychological.[45]

All such issues reflect, at least in part, the bureaucracy and power of institutions that so often foster a sense of helplessness, a sense of us and them (patients), which to the eye of the beholder may easily be interpreted as gender bias. The sense of helplessness of a single mother is tellingly captured in Kim Dayton's story *Procedures.*

One episode begins with the mother being asked by the doctor, 'who was not really a doctor yet', whether she had gone down to the billing office.'

> And I said, 'I think that's already taken care of.'
> 'Well, it says here on the chart that you need to be seen in billing, so perhaps you should go down there now.'
> 'But when will I get to see the baby?'
> And the nurse said, 'They are doing some procedures right now, so it will be a while, so why don't you just go on down to billing, and then go get some rest, and then perhaps everything will be ready and you can see the baby.'
> 'Procedures? What do you mean, procedures?'
> 'Did anyone show you the parents' sleeping room?'
> And I said, 'Yes.'
> Then the doctor said, 'Where is Dad?' and I just looked at him ...
> Then the fat nurse said, 'Mrs. Colson, you will need to leave for a while because we need do some procedures.'
> 'What kind of procedures?' I asked.
> 'Standard procedures.'
> 'Like what?'
> And she said, 'Well, we have to draw some blood, and we have to suction, and weigh her, and so on, and I think it would be best if you just stepped out.'

The mother goes on to relate that she stepped outside, but at least knew where her baby was and was able to watch.[46]

In closing these comments on gender stereotyping, it is easy to think that they apply only to women. However, a general awareness is gathering that beliefs about masculinity 'play a role in shaping male behavioral patterns in ways that have consequences for health.'[47] As with women's health issues, the depth to which these are rooted in culture has always to be appreciated by everyone involved in healthcare. This includes consideration of exactly what is understood by masculinity and masculine ideals, often defined as maintaining distinctiveness from women and embracing independence, self-reliance, strength, robustness and toughness, all of which may encourage body building, asserting sexual power and fostering worries over andropause.[48] Thus men's health – influenced by, for instance, ethnicity, economic status, educational levels and sexual orientation – is as multifaceted as that of women.

This chapter's voices about being caged, stereotyped and classified are but a skimming of the surface of concerns. They have relevance to countless aspects of life in our complex societies, and physicians are being increasingly challenged to consider that, in being empathetic to patients' feelings, they must recognise that these arise not only from the conditions imposed by illness, but also from cultural biases. Physicians are being asked to examine the extent to which a patient's medical and cultural situation may affect their own clinical decision making.

Endnotes

1   Defining normal can be a contentious issue. For one discussion, Davis PV and Bradley JG (1996) The meanings of normal. *Perspectives in Biology and Medicine.* **40**: 68–77.

2   For an example of the caged animal metaphor used by a patient: 'I was ashamed of being mad. This was the 1980s and there was a wall of silence from the medical establishment. I got no help from the doctors. They observed me like a caged animal, watching how my brain worked by making me play scrabble.' (Buckingham C (c. 1997) MindOut for Mental Health: www.mindout.clarity.uk.net/1in4/CB.asp (accessed July 2004). For 'Caged Butterfly', winning essay of Davidson J (c. 2000) for the Mental Health Foundation's Mental Health Week Victorian School Essay Competition for years 10–12: www.depressionet.com.au/articles/butterfly.html (accessed July 2004). For bell-jar metaphor, Plath S (1963) *The Bell Jar.* HarperCollins, London. An autobiographical novel by the celebrated poet.

3   Camus' story allows him to explore broad themes of freedom alongside the duties of a physician.

4   Hospital JT (1983) *The Tiger in the Tiger Pit.* McClelland and Stewart, Toronto, p. 11.

5   Dickey J (1967) 'The Hospital Window'. In his *Poems 1957–1967.* Wesleyan University Press, Middletown. Annotation on poem by Jack Coulehan: www.endeavor.med.nyu.edu/lit-med/lit-med-db/webdocs/webdescrips/dickey220-des-.html (accessed July 2004).

6   For a comprehensive review of differing viewpoints, Couser GT (2001) The cases of Oliver Sacks: the ethics of neuroanthropology. Lecture delivered to Indiana University. www.pointer.Indiana.edu/publications/m-couser.pdf (accessed May 2004).

7   Used here Sacks O (1990) *Awakenings.* Harper Perennial, New York, with a new foreword by Sacks.

8   For useful discussions on the outbreak raising questions about the nature of infectious diseases, Ward CD (1986) Encephalitis lethargica and the development of neuropsychiatry. *Psychiatric Clinics of North America.* **9**: 215–24. The volume of literature was torrential in the 1920s, but became a trickle by the end of the next decade when new cases were rare. See Howard RS and Lees AJ (1987) Encephalitis lethargica: a report of four recent cases. *Brain.* **110**: 19–33.

9   Sacks (1990) *Awakenings*, p. 204.

10   Leonard L from ibid., p. 205.

11   Ibid., p. 207.

12   Ibid., p. 209.

13   Ibid., p. 219.

14   Ibid., pp. 207–8.

15   Bauby J-D (1997) *The Diving Bell and the Butterfly* (English translation). Fourth Estate, London, p. 13. Locked-in syndrome is sometimes discussed in the context of coma, persistent vegetative state and minimal conscious state, but it is sharply different because of its characteristic of full consciousness.

16   Ibid., pp. 11 and 13.

17   Ibid., pp. 61–2.

18   Ibid., p. 90.

19   Treves F (1923) *The Elephant Man and Other Reminiscences.* Cassell, London, pp. 1–37 for various quotes.

20   Noted in Treves F (1885) A case of congenital deformity. *Transactions of the Pathological Society of London.* **36**: 494–8.

21   Buckingham (c. 1997) MindOut for Mental Health.

22   Quote from Andrews J, Briggs A, Porter R *et al.* (1997) *The History of Bethlem.* Routledge, London, p. 178.

23   For expression, Scull A (1993) *The Most Solitary of Afflictions: madness and society in Britain, 1700–1900.* Yale University Press, New Haven.

24   Noted in Hyler SE, Gabbard GO and Schneider I (1991) Homicidal maniacs and narcissistic parasites: stigmatization of mentally ill persons in the movies. *Hospital and Community Psychiatry.* **42**: 1044–8.

25   Gibbons K (1995) *Sights Unseen.* Putnam's Sons, New York.

26 There is no doubt that psychiatry has received far more movie attention than any other medical specialty. In a detailed study, *Psychiatry and the Cinema*, American Psychiatric Press, Washington, 1999, p. xix, Glen Gabbard and Krin Gabbard noted that in the first edition of the book (1986) their filmography depicting psychiatrists was approximately 300 movies, but approached 450 by 1999. Such films have been broadly classified in three groups: Dr Dippy (the comic psychiatrist who could be a patient, ranging from *Dr Dippy's Sanitarium* (1906) to *What About Bob?* (1991)); Dr Evil (the psychopath, the constant abuser of women, or the financially greedy as in *Dressed to Kill*); and Dr Wonderful. See Schneider I (1987) The theory and practice of movie psychiatry. *American Journal of Psychiatry*. **144**: 996–1002. Compared with the Dr Evils, there are relatively few Dr Wonderfuls.

27 For overview, Double DB (2002) History of anti-psychiatry: essay review. *History of Psychiatry*. **13**: 231–6.

28 For an association between, for instance, the concepts of RD Laing and movies, see Hyler, Gabbard and Schneider (1991) Homicidal maniacs and narcissistic parasites: stigmatization of mentally ill persons in the movies. In the 1990s, although psychiatrist Thomas Szsaz's influence as an arch critic of psychiatry had waned substantially since the 1960s, he was still arguing in academic journals. In 1994, he summarised his work over time: 'I have tried to show that the scientific or unscientific character of psychiatry has nothing to do with its abuse. This is because the *professional uses* and *political abuses* of psychiatry are tributaries of the same stream, called 'power'. I maintain that without psychiatric power there could be neither psychiatric abuse nor normal psychiatric practice, as we know it. If mental diseases truly were like other diseases; if the law truly treated mental diseases and mental patients like it treats bodily diseases and ordinary patients; and if psychiatrists truly were like other doctors, then psychiatric practice – like dermatological or ophthalmological practice – would have to be limited to consenting clients (and to children and adults declared legally incompetent).' (Szasz T (1994) Psychiatric diagnosis, psychiatric power and psychiatric abuse. *Journal of Medical Ethics*. **20**: 135–8.)

29 Some of the concerns with psychiatric 'labelling' are to be seen in the context of broad changes, dependent on many factors, in psychiatry over time. On psychosis, as a good example, see Beer MD (1995) Psychosis from mental disorder to disease concept. *History of Psychiatry*. **6**: 177–200.

30 Gabbard and Gabbard (1999) *Psychiatry and the Cinema*, pp. 173–4.

31 Another view is expressed by Schneider I (1987) The theory and practice of movie psychiatry. See also Hyler, Gabbard and Schneider (1991) Homicidal maniacs and narcissistic parasites: stigmatization of mentally ill persons in the movies.

32 Although transference and counter-transference are commonly recognised as a particular hazard of the practice of psychiatry – due to the nature of long-term physician–patient relationships – it is often overlooked as a potential issue in all areas of medicine.

33 We cannot even begin to give a real sense of the pervasiveness, but see issues in relation to psychiatry: Andrews J and Digby A (eds) (2004) *Sex and Seclusion, Class and Custody: perspectives on gender and class in the history of British and Irish psychiatry*. Rodopi, Amsterdam.

34 Chase AW (1862) *Dr Chase's Recipes or Information for Everybody*. AW Chase, Michigan, pp. 189–91.

35 Pierce RV (1914) *The People's Common Sense Adviser*. World's Dispensary Medical Association, Bridgeburg, p. 346.

36 Some of the women have received close attention in recent years such as the fictionalised Alice James in Susan Sontag's play *Alice in Bed*, Farrar, Stauss and Giroux, New York, 1993; also Winter A (1998) A calculus of suffering: Ada Lovelace and the bodily constraints on women's knowledge in early Victorian England. In: Lawrence C and Shapin S (eds) *Science Incarnate: historical embodiments of natural knowledge*. University of Chicago Press, Chicago, pp. 202–39.

37 Jordanova L (1989) *Sexual Visions: images of gender in science and medicine between the eighteenth and twentieth centuries*. University of Wisconsin Press, Madison, p. 96.

38 Cartwright L (1995) *Screening the Body: tracing medicine's visual culture*. University of Minnesota Press, Minneapolis, pp. 146, 147.

39 Yee J (2002) Malaria and the femme fatale: sex and death in French Colonial Africa. *Literature and Medicine*. **21**: 201–15.

40 Gabbard and Gabbard (1999) *Psychiatry and the Cinema*, p. 147. For general discussion of the female psychotherapist in movies, pp. 147–69.

41 Jordanova (1989) *Sexual Visions.* p. 142.

42 The literature on women physicians/healers is substantial. Prejudice is widespread, though not always consistent. Cf. Furst LR (1997) *Women Healers and Physicians: climbing a long hill.* University Press of Kentucky, Lexington. We add a useful website: 'Women Physician's Autobiographies www.research.med.umkc.edu/teams/cml/womendrs.html (accessed June 2004).

43 Dixon LS (1995) *Perilous Chastity: women and illness in pre-enlightenment art and medicine.* Cornell University Press, Ithaca, pp. 243–6. The frequency of images of women in medical advertisements has been studied a number of times. In 1988, one such investigation suggested persistent stereotypes and significant differences between men and women in terms of parts of the body, ethereal, caricature, naked, as spouse, and wearing wedding ring. The study concluded that 'until portrayals of women are consistently positive and timely, the images can have a negative effect on the healthcare women receive.' (Hawkins JW and Aber CS (1988) The content of advertisements in medical journals: distorting the image of women. *Women and Health.* **14** (2): 43–59).

44 Donnison J (1977) *Midwives and Medical Men: a history of inter-professional rivalries and women's rights.* Heinemann, London, and the paperback edition of 1988 with the new subtitle *A History of the Struggle for the Control of Childbirth*, Historical Publications, London, appeared at a time of growing emphasis on natural and holistic health and calls for legalising midwives as a response to the widespread use of drugs in obstetrics and total reliance on physicians.

    Childbirth is only one instance of concerns about the medicalisation of many aspects of women's health; equally well known is premenstrual tension, PMS (or, if serious, labelled as Late Luteal Phase Dysphoric Disorder). At issue again is the question, just what is normal? When, for instance, is PMS a disease rather than a condition? Answers to the question are complicated by many factors. One is encouragement of a disease mindset by PMS clinics, treatment and research. On the other hand, although the term can offer women a welcome medical validation for the condition, it may still be dismissed by male physicians as either imaginary or malingering (its just 'normal' or 'in your head'). Furthermore, some consider that the consequences of a 'medical diagnosis' may be problematic for women overall, since it predisposes menstruating women to be viewed as potential patients at a time when the women's movement places emphasis on women taking control of their bodies.

45 Ballweg ML (1997) Blaming the victim: the psychologizing of endometriosis. *Obstetrics and Gynecology Clinics of North America.* **24**: 441–53.

46 Dayton K (1999) Procedures. In: Haddad AM and Brown KH (eds) *The Arduous Touch: women's voices in health care.* NotaBell Books, West Lafayette, pp. 12–20.

47 Williams DR (2003) The health of men: structured inequalities and opportunities. *American Journal of Public Health.* **93**: 724–31.

48 E.g. Courtenay WH (2000) Constructions of masculinity and their influence on men's well-being: a theory of gender and health. *Social Science and Medicine.* **50**: 1385–401.

CHAPTER 11

Physicians' approaches to disease

This chapter, after first looking at the heart as a cultural symbol, turns more directly to concepts internal to medicine that can affect a physician's approach to disease. Earlier considerations on decision making are expanded by focusing more specifically on medical thinking. Many people wonder how two practitioners can be led to different decisions – at least in details – about the same patient's treatment regimen. Although the illustrations in this chapter focus mainly on cardiovascular matters, analogous issues are common to all specialty areas of medicine.

The heart as a pump and cultural symbol

The heart, more than any other organ, is surrounded by deeply held cultural beliefs. These not only provide pitfalls for miscommunication between physicians and patients, but also raise again the issue of reductionism considered in Chapter 4.

An ever-lingering question concerning the heart is whether it is to be viewed merely as a pump. Although the question emerged with William Harvey's discovery of the circulation of the blood (1628) and his later analogy of the heart to a mechanical pump, it was only with the first heart transplantation in 1967 that public debate focused on whether or not the heart is the seat of the emotions. Philip Blaiberg vigorously expressed one view in 1968:

> Today I am the second man since the Creation to live with the heart of a dead man beating in his breast, able to declare that the heart is not the seat of the emotions, of love and hate, good and evil, greed and generosity; to prove it as a pump that can wear out or be damaged and, like a car part, replaced to continue the task of powering the engine of the body.[1]

In the same year, Peter Medawar, the eminent biologist and Nobel Laureate whose work on immunology helped to set the stage for heart transplantation, accurately predicted: 'The transplantation of human organs will be assimilated into ordinary clinical practice ... and there will be no need to be philosophical about it. This will come about for the single and sufficient reason that people are so constituted that they would be rather alive than dead.'[2]

In the light of the intense ethical/philosophical debate that surrounded the first human heart transplant, it is of particular interest that no reference to issues surrounding the emotions or ethics (e.g. on how to ensure the donor was dead and on whether black hearts should be transplanted into white people) appeared in the 1969 autobiography of Christiaan Barnard, the South African surgeon who performed the first and second transplants.[3] Barnard dealt essentially with medical aspects of the operation and the tremendous fight to save the life of Louis Washkansky, the first transplant patient, who died after eight days.[4] It is not altogether surprising, then, that in recent years little public debate on the relationship between the heart and the soul has been evident; certainly relevant has been acceptance of heart transplants by major religions in the West.[5] There is also general acceptance of the development of the artificial heart, even though the 'success' of implantations up to 2004 is debatable.[6] Such a trend can be viewed as one more way in which medical technology has become an integral part of the specialty of cardiology. Indeed, cardiologists are sometimes stereotyped as primarily technicians who measure pressures in the chambers of the heart, look for blockages in the coronary circulation with dyes and X-rays, prescribe pacemakers, monitor cardiac and blood pressure with oscilloscopes, and so on.

Yet, despite attitudes suggestive that ideas of the heart as the mysterious seat of the soul and the emotions have been moved to the cultural backstage, diverse factors continue to sustain it as a cultural symbol and metaphor; such factors range from the well-known physiological impact of emotions on the circulatory system to 'messages' that the heart is 'our emotional and spiritual life force'[7] (cf. also Box 11.1). Many such messages are embedded in popular culture. For instance, the movie *Heart Condition* (1990) centres around a bigoted white cop who receives a transplant from an African-American along with his ghost (or is it his soul?). A contrasting example of the pervasiveness of cultural symbolism can be found in the memoirs of Eva Salber, a 'physician/scientist/humanist', which describe her work among the poor and underserved people in South Africa, Boston and rural North Carolina. Two verses in the book's preface are indicative as to why Salber remains a role model for physicians years after her death.[8]

> The mind – is not the heart.
> I may yet live, as I know others live,
> To wish in vain to let go with the mind –
> Of cares, at night, to sleep; but nothing tells me
> That I need learn to let go with the heart.
>
> Robert Frost
>
> What is knowledge
> Without the intrinsic mediation of the heart?
>
> RP Warren

Box 11.1 'You'll find Jesus there'

The following story circulated on the Internet in 2001. Clearly it was intended to provide comfort to those who know dying children, but it also prompts thoughts on how many people attribute non-pump roles to the heart.

'Tomorrow morning,' the surgeon began, 'I'll open up your heart ...'

'You'll find Jesus there,' the boy interrupted.

The surgeon looked up, annoyed 'I'll cut your heart open,' he continued, 'to see how much damage has been done ... '

'But when you open up my heart, you'll find Jesus in there.'

The surgeon looked to the parents, who sat quietly.

'When I see how much damage has been done, I'll sew your heart and chest back up and I'll plan what to do next.'

'But you'll find Jesus in my heart. The Bible says He lives there. The hymns all say He lives there. You'll find Him in my heart.'

The surgeon had had enough. 'I'll tell you what I'll find in your heart. I'll find damaged muscle, low blood supply, and weakened vessels. And I'll find out if I can make you well.'

'You'll find Jesus there too. He lives there.'

The surgeon left.

The surgeon sat in his office, recording his notes from the surgery, '... damaged aorta, damaged pulmonary vein, widespread muscle degeneration. No hope for transplant, no hope for cure.'

'Therapy: painkillers and bed rest.'

'Prognosis:' Here he paused 'Death within one year.'

He stopped the recorder, but there was more to be said.

'Why?' he asked aloud. 'Why did You do this? You've put him here; you've put him in this pain; and You've cursed him to an early death. Why?'

The Lord answered and said, 'The Boy, My lamb, was not meant for your flock for long, for he is a part of My flock, and will forever be. Here, in My flock, he will feel no pain, and will be comforted as you cannot imagine. His parents will one day join him here, and they will know peace, and My flock will continue to grow.'

The surgeon's tears were hot, but his anger was hotter. 'You created that boy, and You created that heart. He'll be dead in months. Why?'

The Lord answered, 'The boy, My lamb, shall return to My flock, for he has done his duty: I did not put My lamb with your flock to lose him, but to retrieve another lost lamb.'

The surgeon wept.

The surgeon sat beside the boy's bed; the boy's parents sat across from him. The boy awoke and whispered, 'Did you cut open my heart?'

'Yes,' said the surgeon.

'What did you find?' asked the boy.

'I found Jesus there,' said the surgeon.

Author unknown

There are, too, countless examples of physicians who, while feeling that little mystery remains about the heart, express deep reverence for it. None speaks more evocatively than Richard Selzer when writing on the anatomical intricacies of the heart. For instance, that 'the lining of each cavity is thrown up into folds, or trabeculations, that would seem to be organic responses to the jet and turbulence of the blood. The upper portions of these chambers are strung with a tracery of fine, fibrous cords that go from the muscle of the heart to the cusps of the valves, holding them in place like tent ropes. These corda tendinea have none of the brawn of the ventricles but are delicate strings that seem made for the blood to fret upon.'[9]   We leave thoughts of the heart as a cultural symbol by asking whether they contribute unconsciously to the reluctance of many people to sign organ donor cards, or to families 'vetoing' organ donation by loved ones.[10] Do many people have lurking doubts about whether the heart is solely a pump, even if they do not voice such thoughts with their doctors? After the death of one patient following implantation of the AbioCor artificial heart, the wife, knowing that the heart would be returned to the manufacturer for study, requested that the surgeon find whatever was left of the original heart and to replace it in the chest. In death, the wife wanted her husband to have a 'human heart'.[11]

Disease concepts and dichotomies

The paradoxical concepts of the heart as both a pump and as the seat of the emotions (i.e. mechanical *and* non-mechanical roles) reflects, in a very loose sense, a general dichotomy in ways of approaching disease, namely either reductionist or holistic; this, as will be noted, can have potential implications in clinical practice.

Remarks such as 'there's a classical Tay-Sachs in 219C', typically heard among hospital staff, unwittingly echo an essential contradiction that has characterised medical theory and practice for 2000 years: is there really a disease that is a 'discrete entity', as if it could exist outside the body?[12] The notion of a discrete disease entity has been encouraged over time by, for instance, concepts that see the body as analogous to a machine, or others that place emphasis on the localisation of pathology to specific organs; the latter concept was developed fully in the nineteenth century supported by new diagnostic tools for physical examinations; relevant, too, were new theories such as germs causing disease, and concepts of chemotherapy and specificity in therapy already noted in Chapter 9.

It is confusing, perhaps, that other terms also describe, or at least substantially overlap, the notion of a 'disease entity'. One is 'form', which implies specific pathological lesions; form, it must be noted, is usually paired with the contrary term 'function' to describe disease as being essentially a change in bodily functions. A corollary of this is to view disease as a disorder of a *system* that produces a range of symptoms. Such a dichotomy – form/function – is virtually synonymous with other pairs of terms such as ontological/physiological. Ontology is another term referring to diseases as specific entities independent of how they are manifest in individual patients. A physiological viewpoint, on the other hand, often viewed as a 'holistic' approach, tends to see a patient's sickness as specific to that individual.[13] The latter is covered by yet another term 'clinical entity', often used in the context of practitioners responding to and taking care of *all* of a particular patient's signs and symptoms as well as specific personal concerns and worries.

The existence of all of these terms is not to say that hard and fast dichotomies are the norm in everyday practice. However, *tendencies* to approach disease in terms of a disease entity opens the door for a practitioner, indeed likely predisposes him or her, to a mindset of a war on disease (cf. Chapter 9); moreover, it may foster tendencies to ignore, even dismiss as irrelevant, symptoms identified by a patient that do not match those listed in textbook diagnoses. It can also mean pushing to one side the very issues – spiritual, for instance – on which patients want help. A clinical or functional mindset, on the other hand, as said, fosters emphasis on caring for the entire spectrum of a patient's symptoms and worries. It can mean more ready acceptance of such conditions as chronic fatigue syndrome as a 'real problem' whereas, in the absence of an accepted aetiology for an eclectic range of symptoms, some physicians may continue to dismiss a patient's symptoms as 'all in the mind'. Within cardiology a functional mindset may foster greater readiness to explore the complexity of lifestyles to deal with cardiovascular disease. After all cardiology has come to see 'excesses' as a primary aetiology – excesses of diet, smoking, of leisure without exercise – along with resistance to change to healthier lifestyles.

The extent to which physicians are predisposed to see disease as a discrete entity not only varies from physician to physician and over time, but also from specialty to specialty. The notes that follow on four examples illuminate subtleties that have shaped physician care, or have the potential to continue to do so.

Although many physicians with a special interest in cardiology shifted in mindset from concepts of localised pathology to physiological explanations for certain diseases in the late nineteenth and early twentieth centuries, this was soon to change again. The growth in acceptance of such concepts as atherosclerosis (as a cause of coronary thrombosis) and the use of quantitative measurements (e.g. for defining hypertension) returned cardiological mindsets to disease entities between 1910 and 1930. Then, it has been argued, functional notions were pushed aside in the cardiological literature. For instance, although medical textbooks at the time still stated that tachycardia could be caused by 'nervousness' or 'neurosis', heart specialists defined it as falling outside the relatively new specialist discipline of cardiology; rather, such cases were to be treated as psychiatric.[14]

The history of angina pectoris is especially noteworthy for its shift, around the 1930s, from being seen as a protean condition – it straddled being viewed as a disease and a clinical entity – to a disease entity alone, at least as viewed by leaders of the then growing specialty of cardiology. They excluded from cardiology any chest pain that could not be diagnosed as due to diseased coronary arteries and hence no longer diagnosed as angina. A new breed of heart specialists were thus defining their field to cover only demonstrably organic and pathophysiological disorders, a shift that aided the development of cardiology as a distinct medical specialty.[15]

The pain of angina pectoris is classically linked to exertion (occasioning a shortage of oxygen reaching the cardiac muscle). By the 1930s, as already indicated, the condition was widely accepted as being due to atherosclerotic blockage. It is tempting to suggest that this view contributed to the failure to give serious consideration to alternative explanations to blockage as the cause of the pain such as it being due to spasm of the coronary arteries. After all, it was recognised that anginal pain was quite variable, including occurring at rest. In 1959, Myron Prinzmetal and colleagues argued that the latter (pain at rest) should be viewed as a distinct entity – it came to be known as Prinzmetal's angina, variant angina pectoris or unstable angina pectoris. In noting that 'cases are not diagnosed for several reasons' they recognised a conceptual mindset, that of blockage, hindered alternative views.[16] Although spasm of the coronary vessels had been suggested as an aetiology as early as 1941, it was not until 1973 (following improved X-ray visualisation techniques) that the physiological explanation was confirmed, namely that spontaneous spasm in an *anatomically normal* coronary artery could produce angina.[17]

To reinforce a point, it is useful to note that, in contrast to classifying angina pectoris as a disease rather than a clinical entity, perceptions of kidney disease were shifting the other way around the 1920s and '30s. This is reflected in the changing 'labels' for kidney failure: from dropsy (whether this was due to kidney or heart disease was not differentiated until the nineteenth century) to Bright's disease, and then such terms as glomerulonephritis, renal failure and end-stage renal disease. Such changes also underscore how names of diseases conjure particular fears and responses, and asks the question whether the current term, end-stage renal disease, is helpful. As one patient has said, 'it sounds like the end of the world.'[18] It leaves dangling the role of hope that many practitioners feel is a necessary part of a treatment regimen.

Another condition, over which each physician should consciously consider whether his or her attitudes to disease may shape their management of patients, is essential hypertension. Over time, the diversity of attitudes towards the condition provide for a particularly fascinating history. By the 1930s various considerations fostered acceptance of essential hypertension as a specific disease entity, despite it being a condition without any consensus as to its cause. The influence of leaders of the medical profession such as T Clifford Allbutt was significant, aided by speculative theories that cast it as having specific, localised pathology.[19] There was, too, the seductiveness of technology (the sphygmomanometer) that allowed all physicians to monitor blood pressure regularly. Moreover, at the time, renowned cardiologist Paul Dudley White authoritatively promoted precise quantitative limits for 'normal' blood pressure. He wrote (1931) in his standard textbook on the heart: 'the extreme normal limits for the systolic blood pressure of the adult at rest are 95 and 145 millimeters of mercury, regardless of age or size, but a narrower range of 110 to 130 millimeters is more usual.'[20] He also emphasised the importance of diastolic blood pressure, giving normal adult limits of between 60 and 90 millimetres. 'If it is abnormally high it means excessive constant strain for the circulation.' Accepted limits of 90/140 (later revised) gave a sense of precision, a sense of a specific disease to be treated. This view became firmly cemented in place with the availability of an increasing number of *specific* treatments (contrasting with the more general action of diuretics) emerging in the second half of the twentieth century.

There has, however, been constant debate as to whether essential hypertension should be seen as a disease, albeit a 'silent' disease. A celebrated debate between two renowned British physicians, Lord Platt and Sir George Pickering, argued the issue for 20 years or so. In essence, Platt saw it as a disease entity; Pickering, on the other hand, viewed it as a clinical entity; unlike Platt, he did not consider inheritance an overriding factor in the aetiology, but argued that essential hypertension was multifactorial.[21] By and large the latter view has prevailed, although some prefer to view essential hypertension as a 'risk factor'.[22] A 1990 review of hypertension remains a succinct summary of the argument that treatment must always be approached on the basis that individuals vary one from another.

> The bulk of the evidence still favours the view that hypertension is a heterogeneous process, with different mechanisms dominant in different individuals. As such, attempts to identify a single abnormality that separates normotensive and hypertensive individuals are unlikely to succeed ... the natural history is also variable, because it is only a minority of patients who suffer any ill effects from their blood pressure. Consequently, a rigid stepped-care approach to the hypertensive patient is to be deplored. The onus on the physician is to take into consideration each patient's entire clinical picture and to assess the relative contributions of different underlying mechanisms. The decision to treat should be based on the evaluation of risk, not simply on the level of blood pressure measured in the clinic; and finally, it should be remembered that the goal of treatment is not to lower blood pressure but to lower morbidity.[23]

Notwithstanding such views, many physicians continue to emphasise medication rather than concentrating on changing lifestyles.

One lifestyle regimen – the Dean Ornish approach to combat or treat atherosclerosis – serves as our last example in which a disease mindset in cardiology may affect decision making. Despite evidence published in conventional peer review journals that the diet (the key part of a regimen that comprises a very low fat diet along with non-smoking, stress reduction, yoga and exercise) can reverse coronary heart disease and so avoid angioplasty or bypass surgery, Ornish's approach has received relatively little attention among professionals as a non-invasive alternative.[24] The question to be asked is whether a key reason relates to beliefs that existing approaches – surgical to remove blockage and drug treatment (e.g. cholesterol-lowering drugs) – fit more closely with war on disease (Chapter 9) or patients' demands for immediate relief. In contrast, Ornish's approach is a lengthy one – a functional one – that demands a commitment to marked changes in lifestyles. Indeed, much of the tepid reception to Ornish, such as from the American Heart Association, is belief that the discipline required to maintain the diet is beyond the will-power of most people.

A dilemma for patients, as noted at the beginning of this chapter, is conflicting medical opinions. Such dilemmas can be heightened when one physician criticises another. Patients need to appreciate more than just the uncertainties that continue to surround the outcomes of disease; they also need some understanding of the nature of medical thinking, of medical mindsets. In turn, the medical profession as a whole must ask itself about its responsibility to help develop such an understanding.

Endnotes

1   Blaiberg P (1968) *Looking at My Heart*. Stein and Day, New York, p. 15.
2   Quoted in Anyanwu A and Treasure T (2003) Prognosis after heart transplantation. *British Medical Journal*. **326**: 509–10.
3   Barnard C and Pepper CB (1970) *Christiaan Barnard, One Life*. Macmillan, Toronto. Later, Barnard stated: 'We didn't see the heart as the seat of soul. The cessation of the heart did not mean the end of life. We knew that.' Quoted in 'Thirtieth Anniversary of Heart

Transplants' (BBC News): www.news.bbc.co.uk/1/hi/sci/tech/36604.stm (accessed July 2004). Some discussion of ethical issues raised over heart transplantation appear in Rothman DJ (1991) *Strangers at the Bedside: a history of how law and bioethics transformed medical decision making*. Basic Books, New York, pp. 156–9, 165–7.

4   Barnard and Pepper (1970) *Christiaan Barnard, One Life*, pp. 321–87 for an account of Washkansky's 18 days of post-operative care; one author has said that a layman reading the account of Washkansky's last days 'may react as one does to human torture.' (Wertenbaker L (1980) *To Mend the Heart*. Viking Press, New York, p. 210.)

5   The story of the artificial heart is an intriguing one of expectations of success marred by relatively short survival times of patients due to strokes and infections. Amid the substantial literature, a short discussion by F Gil (1989) of political ethical issues is still relevant: The artificial heart juggernaut. *Hastings Center Report*. March/April: 24–31.

6   Fox RC and Swazey JP (2004) in 'He knows that machine in his mortality'. Old and new social and cultural patterns in the clinical trial of the AbioCor artificial heart. *Perspectives in Biology and Medicine*. **47**: 74–99, point out that, while claims have been made for the success of the AbioCor artificial heart, the quality of life until death of the patients with the heart prompts questions about how to define 'success'. Answering such a question is made more difficult by the aura of pioneering and heroism that has been erected around the implantation players, both patients and surgeons. The issue is media publicity, and for a useful discussion on media and medicine with the AbioCor heart as an example, Morreim EH (2004) High-profile research and the media: the case of the AbioCor artifical heart. *Hastings Center Report*. January/February: 11–24.

7   Marks L and Lee D 'Healing the Heart, Reaching the Soul: the neurobiology of body-centered psychotherapy': www.ahpweb.org/pub/perspective/heart.html (accessed July 2004). Bennett H and Sparrow S (no date) 'The Thinking Heart: an interview with Paul Pearsall': www.ikosmos.com/wisdomeditions/essays/mw/bennett01.htm (accessed July 2004). The latter argues that transplant patients who receive an organ donor from another person's body may also receive what Pearsall calls their 'cellular memories'. Recipients, it is said, have reported inheriting everything from the donor's food cravings to knowledge about murder.

8   Salber EJ (1989) *The Mind is Not the Heart: recollections of a woman physician*. Duke University Press, Durham, pp. ix and xiv. The account, and her earlier book *Don't Send Me Flowers When I'm Dead* (1983), reveals why Salber had a reputation as an empathic physician who continues to serve as a role model years after her death in 1991.

9   Selzer R (1995) The surgeon as writer. In: Penney JC (ed) *Proceedings of the Humanities Conference at Dalhousie Medical School, February 7–9, 1991*. Faculty of Medicine, Dalhousie Medical School, Halifax, pp. 56–63. Selzer's account follows remarks on the death and autopsy of his father.

10 Transplantation, of course, raises countless concerns as evidenced in popular culture. For instance, the movie *Coma* (1978), based on a novel by Robin Cook, remains well known for focusing attention on the black market in transplanted organs. A more recent movie example is *Donor Unknown* (1995), based on the novel *Corazon* by William Mooney.

11 See Fox and Swazey (2004) 'He Knows that Machine in his Mortality'.

12 Comment from Hudson RP (1983) *Disease and its Control: the shaping of modern thought*. Greenwood Press, Westport, p. 229 *et seq.*

13 Cf. Aronowitz RA (1998) *Making Sense of Illness: science, society, and disease*. Cambridge University Press, Cambridge, p. 8.

14 Lawrence C (1992) Coronary thrombosis and cardiologists. In: Rosenberg C and Golden J (eds) *Framing Disease: studies in cultural history*. Rutgers University Press, New Brunswick, pp. 50–82.

15 Cf. ibid. and Aronowitz (1998) From the patient's angina pectoris to the cardiologist's coronary heart disease. In his *Making Sense of Illness: science, society, and disease*, pp. 84–110.

16 Prinzmetal M, Kennamer R, Merliss R *et al.* (1959) Angina pectoris l. A variant form of angina pectoris. *American Journal of Medicine*. **27**: 375–88.

17 Oliva PB, Potts DE and Pluss RG (1973) Coronary arterial spasm in Prinzmetal angina: documentation by coronary arteriography. *New England Journal of Medicine*. **288**: 745–51.

18 Peitzman SJ (1992) From Bright's disease to end-stage renal disease. In: Rosenberg and Golden (eds) *Framing Disease: studies in cultural history*, pp. 3–19.

19 Allbutt, of national and international renown, had a special interest in arterial disease and blood pressure. To emphasise his view that essential hypertension was a distinct entity he introduced the term 'hyperpiesia'. However, it was E Frank's alternative term 'essentielle hypertonie' that became generally accepted. For some of Allbutt's mature views, see his *Arteriosclerosis: a summary view*. Macmillian, London, 1925.

20 White PD (1931) *Heart Disease*. Macmillan, New York, pp. 131–2. See also his interesting comments on normal blood pressures in White PD (1971) *My Life and Medicine: an autobiographical memoir*. Gambit, Boston, pp. 107–8.

21 For the debate, Swales JD (ed) (1985) *Platt versus Pickering: an episode in recent medical history*. Keynes Press/British Medical Association, London.

22 The view that essential hypertension was best viewed as a risk factor rather than a disease emerged in the 1980s. Cf. Kawachi I and Wilson N (1990) The evolution of antihypertensive therapy. *Social Science and Medicine*. **31**: 1239–43.

23 Pickering TG (1990) Afterword to Chapter 1 (written by Sir George Pickering). In: Laragh JH and Brenner BM (eds) *Hypertension, Pathology, Diagnosis and Management*, vol. 1. Raven Press, New York, pp. 17–19.

24 Rather than reference Ornish's scientific papers, note the 2002 article Dean Ornish, MD: a conversation with the editor. *American Journal of Cardiology*. **90**: 271–98. This offers some insight, at least from one point of view, to the many issues surrounding Ornish's efforts to introduce new approaches to treatment.

Physician and patient responsibilities

The loudness of the public voice in recent years – its hopes and expectations with regard to medical care – suggests that, nowadays, individual physicians have to earn their public respect. No longer can even the local family practitioner rely on riding, as it were, on the prestigious coat-tails of the medical profession as a whole. Many physicians, as indicated in various places in this volume, must now be aware how readily public opinion can shift. What happened to Doc Meyers in the *Spoon River Anthology* (noted in Chapter 2) is a local story that, even though bound in time and place, has a universal message for today. Recently, a past president of the British General Medical Council has written: 'Public confidence in a profession is sustained when its expectations are – or are perceived to be – in harmony with professional culture and performance. On the other hand, public confidence is undermined when a significant gap appears between general expectation and performance. This is what happened to the medical profession in the later years of the 20th century.'[1]

To the voices in this volume, one can add countless others, some only heard locally. For instance, Melissa Goldstein, suffering from systemic lupus erythematosus, tells of offering her rheumatologist her poems to read. Although she received minimal response from him, he distributed them among hospital staff. It later became clear that the poems served as a means of communication and helped to establish Goldstein's role in her own healthcare: 'Eight years after becoming ill, the integration of my writing and my medical care seems entirely natural to me. Throughout my medical chart, one finds my poems and even an essay.'[2]

Reflected in such stories, and in all the voices quoted in this volume, is the need for health practitioners to respond to a changing society and to specific issues such as giving or offering the patient a much bigger role in decision making than in the past: to respect their autonomy.

At the same time, many voices from within medical humanities prompt the public to consider their own roles and responsibilities in healthcare, responsibilities linked to the new autonomy. While much medical commentary continues to centre on the responsibility of patient 'compliance' and on following institutional rules (often posted on websites), greater challenges for patients come from the new 'fountains' of information, mostly from the Internet. The challenges include the need to *understand* the information, even if it is delivered clearly, given the many uncertainties that surround the care and prognosis of illness. Moreover, many people do not find it easy to dialogue with 'experts', even those who have the ability to communicate and empathise with a patient. There may, too, be ethical dilemmas to deal with such as when physicians find their clinical judgment limited by institutional and insurance company policies and restrictions.

The whole arena of patients' responsibilities has growing visibility. There is, for instance, the British government initiative, *The Expert Patient: a new approach to chronic disease management for the 21st century*.[3] In noting that the 'era of the patient as a passive recipient of care is changing and being replaced by a new emphasis on the relationship between the [National Health Service] and the people whom it serves', the government initiative involves developing formal programmes in which tutors, who themselves suffer from a relevant chronic ailment such as manic depression or multiple sclerosis, will teach and help others to manage the disease.[4]

An important question, certainly for patients, that arises from such trends is how accepting are physicians of greater involvement by patients, especially as it can lead to time-consuming questions if not new demands. In fact, very diverse physician views exist. They include significant signs of resistance. One survey reported that only 21 per cent of doctors were in favour of the British government's proposals on the Expert Patient.[5] For many physicians the expert patient is the demanding patient, the unreasonable patient, the time-consuming patient, or the patient who knows it all.[6] On the other hand, some physicians are more accepting of terms alternative to expert such as 'autonomous', 'resourceful' or 'involved'. Only some are comfortable with the approach of 'let us learn about your problem together', which fits with other voices that call for therapeutic relationships, with underpinnings of mutual trust and respect so often demanded by patients.[7] It is not unreasonable to suggest that only the latter see acceptance of the new patient demands as part of what might be aptly called a 'new' professionalism.

Public Expectations and Physicians' Responsibilities underscores that public scrutiny and accountability – extending to all walks of life in modern societies – is very much part of modern healthcare. The question arises whether the responses that the profession has already made are sufficient. After all concerns, within and outside the medical profession, about physician roles show no sign of abating. One physician, after considering portrayals of doctors in art, literature and medicine, said recently: 'And if, in the depiction of our trade, perceptions of our benignity and those of our power have been locked in a dispiritingly inverse relationship, what, if anything, can be done?'[9] The author suggests, 'Still wielding our modern wonders, should we not now look backwards too, learn from the great Victorians, cultivate presence and consideration in all levels, and mend our bedside manners.'

Many voices from the public would agree, but this volume makes clear that the responses need to be broader than just looking backwards in the hope of restoring what are perceived to be traditional values associated with a moral character.[10] As made clear in Chapter 2, professionalism has also to ensure that it fits current perceptions in the eyes of its beholders. Individual physicians and professional institutions must recognise societal changes and the notion of a social contract that is generally felt to exist between medicine and the society it serves, and the need for public dialogue about current needs.[11]

At the same time, the public has to recognise that its expectations of physicians cannot be met by all, indeed perhaps by relatively few. It has also to try to understand the biases and inherent uncertainties in medicine. Moreover, the public, with its new autonomy, has to appreciate its responsibilities to debate with the medical profession the structures of and compromises within our healthcare systems – in many ways the result of ad hoc growth – so that healthcare practitioners can fulfil as many patients' wishes and needs as possible.

Endnotes

1   Irvine D (2003) *The Doctors' Tale: professionalism and public trust.* Radcliffe Medical Press, Oxford, pp. 5–6. Irvine places emphasis on technical competencies, but, clearly, public expectations and concerns over trust are of broader concern as indicated in this volume.

2   Goldstein G (1997) Medicine and poetry: a pathway of communication. *The Pharos.* Spring: 12–14.

3   The report, 'The Expert Patient: a new approach to chronic disease management for the 21st century', is available at www.ohn.gov.uk/ohn/people/ep_report.pdf (accessed July 2004).

4   Quote from Executive Summary. Ibid., p. 9.

5   Quoted in Shaw J and Baker M (2004) 'Expert patient': dream or nightmare? *British Medical Journal*, **328**: 723–4.

6   Ibid.

7   For alternative terms to 'expert patient', ibid. Also, for a variety of views, 'Rapid responses': www.bmj.bmjjournals.com/cgi/eletters/328/7442/723 (accessed July 2004). For calls for therapeutic relationships, cf. Crellin JK (2004) *A Social History of Medicines in the Twentieth Century.* Haworth Press, New York, pp. 243–6.

8   Douglas C (2002) Doing better, looking worse. *British Medical Journal.* **325**: 720.

9   Historians have emphasised that a good moral character was seen to be a requisite for physician behaviour up to the twentieth century. E.g. Gidney RD and Miller WPJ (1994) *Professional Gentlemen: the professions in nineteenth-century Ontario.* University of Toronto Press, Toronto.

10 Widespread acceptance of the notion of a social contract is noted in a recent discussion on a working definition of profession with respect to medicine: Creuss SR, Johnston S and Creuss RL (2004) 'Profession': a working definition for medical educators. *Teaching and Learning in Medicine.* **16**: 74–6. However, the discussion does not provide a sense that professionalism must embrace an awareness of change and the need to respond.

Index